Expert endorsements for *Zest for Life*

"As an integrative oncologist, I firmly believe in the importance of consuming as many anti-cancer foods as possible in our diet. Zest for Life is an excellent reference for anyone who wants to learn about how the foods we eat contribute to our overall health and the prevention of cancer.

Conner Middelmann-Whitney is an inspirational Mediterranean diet expert and chef. The pages of her book are filled with passion, clarity, and fun. This is a fantastic reference for my patients, and so well-written that it should be easy for everyone to follow. With enthusiasm, I highly recommend Zest for Life."

Brian Lawenda M.D., integrative oncologist at 21st Century Oncology,
Las Vegas, Nevada; www.integrativeoncology-essentials.com

"Zest for Life follows the tenets of an anti-cancer diet and provides practical and tasty ways of increasing our intake of plant-based whole foods. It is essential that we move toward a plant-based diet, and Zest for Life is a useful book for nutritional education and healthful recipes."

Lorenzo Cohen, Ph.D., Professor and Director of the Integrative Medicine
Program at MD Anderson Cancer Center, Houston, Texas

"A key message of Zest for Life is that the Mediterranean diet is more than the sum of its parts. It includes cultural and lifestyle aspects that favorably affect the risk of several cancers, but also have wider implications on our health. Overweight and obesity, for instance, have not increased in France or Italy over the last three decades, and this has wider implications than cancer risk."

Carlo La Vecchia, Professor of Epidemiology,
school of Medicine, University of Milan; www.marionegri.it

"There are thousands of recipe books advertizing mouth-watering meals with glossy photographs. Zest for Life is not an enticement for succulent cuisine through glossy pictures. It is much better.

Zest for Life teaches you basic science-based principles of nutrition and leads you through some delicious recipes. Follow the recipes – you will have fun and feel healthy. What's more, your family will thank you for it: they will embrace meals as part of life and realize that life is part of meals."

Professor Stephen Sagar, Department of Oncology,
McMaster University; www.stephensagar.com

"More than a cookbook, Zest for Life *is an indispensable guide to the many powerful health benefits of the Mediterranean diet. The food is anti-inflammatory, nutrient-rich and delicious. Definitely worth the effort to prepare. I recommend* Zest for Life *to cancer patients I coach."*

"People affected by cancer need guidance on what foods to eat and how to prepare these healthy food options. Unfortunately there are very few resources that support this need. Conner Middelmann-Whitney approaches this topic in a practical way in Zest for Life, *a wonderful guide for people looking to enhance their nutrition as a tool to increase their defenses against cancer.*

As an integrative physician providing practical advice to patients and families affected by cancer about healthy options that they can integrate in their care, I see this book as a great resource for information and help in addressing some of the nutritional questions that patients bring."

"I recommend this book to everyone, particularly for those with a strong family history of cancer. But following the author's recommendations would do more than lower your risk of cancer. You'd likely have a longer lifespan, lose some excess fat weight, and lower your risk of type 2 diabetes, dementia, heart disease, stroke, obesity, and vision loss from macular degeneration. Particularly compared to the standard American diet. What are you waiting for? Let's get cookin'!"

"Zest for Life *provides discovery and learning critical to understanding why poor eating habits may lead to cancer and is so logical in its content that you'll have one of those "Oh, my gosh"-moments as you realize it makes so much sense.*

These are the most common excuses we hear in our medical practice: "I don't know what to buy," "I don't have the time to get all of that stuff and fix it," or "I can't afford to eat healthy foods." Conner Middelmann-Whitney will help debunk these common myths, and will touch your heart and stimulate the inner-you; the part of you that secretly wants to be healthy, wants to live a long and prosperous life and wants your family to be just as lucky."

Zest for Life

THE MEDITERRANEAN ANTI-CANCER DIET

*A guide to dietary cancer prevention
with over 150 recipes*

Conner Middelmann-Whitney

Honeybourne Publishing

This publication contains the opinions and ideas of its author. It is intended to provide helpful and informative material on the subjects addressed in the publication. It is sold with the understanding that the author is not engaged in rendering medical, health or any other kind of personal or professional services in the book. If the reader requires personal medical, health or other assistance or advice, a competent health professional should be consulted.

Although every care and precaution has been taken in the preparation of this book, the author and publisher specifically disclaim all responsibility for any liability, loss or risk, personal or otherwise, that is incurred as a consequence, directly or indirectly, of the use and application of any of the contents of this book.

Before undertaking significant dietary or lifestyle changes, including a weight-loss plan, or beginning or modifying an exercise program, check with your doctor if these changes are right for you.

Honeybourne Publishing Ltd
Level 2
1 Sun Street
London EC2A 2EP

ISBN 978-0-9568665-0-9

A catalogue record for this book is available from the British Library.

Editors: Colleen Dawson, Glenn Whitney, Anke Middelmann
Cover and content design: John Hawkins, John Hawkins Design (www.jhbd.co.uk)
Cover photograph: Natalia Klenova 2010, used under license from Shutterstock.com
Author photograph: Kurt Witcher, Studio Illume, Toulouse (www.studioillume.com)

Contents

For Glenn, Oscar, Max and Charlotte,
my favourite dining companions

Acknowledgments

My deepest gratitude goes to my mother Hanna and her mother Christel, who not only taught me how to cook but also how to revel in simple, tasty, home-cooked fare and to delight in feeding others. I also thank my father, Wolf, for his love of conviviality, garlic and red wine. Heartfelt thanks go to Mimi for her Mediterranean good cheer and culinary inspiration.

Warm thanks go to all those who believed in this project and supported me in troubled times. I am indebted to my crack team of editors, the eagle-eyed Colleen Dawson, Glenn Whitney, Anke Middelmann and Lucy West, for making this book readable, and to John Hawkins for his endless patience.

Many thanks go to Lybi Ma for inviting me to blog on cancer prevention for *Psychology Today*, to Pascale Hervieux for translations and advice, and to Kim and Tracy Chevalier and Tim Nash for recipe-testing and moral support. Heartfelt thanks also to Richenda Carey, Jeanine Beck, Tina and Andrew Mendelsohn, Ross Tieman, David and Lauren Meisels, Ken Whitney (creator of the *Sardinade*), Cathy Filipowicz, Wiebke Middelmann, Sue Whitney-Wolfson, Francoise Boucek, Laura and Michael van der Sande, Béatrice Grunmeier and Adrian Laing and my dear friends who forgave me my long silences while I was working on this project. Thanks also go to my nutrition clients and cooking-class pupils for their enthusiasm and perseverance; I hope this book may help them on their path of nutritional health and healing.

Profound gratitude goes to the experts who took the time to help me gain a deeper understanding of the link between food and cancer. They include Professor Bharat Aggarwal at the University of Texas M. D. Anderson Cancer Center; Professor Denis Corpet at the University of Toulouse; Dr. Mario Ferruzzi at Purdue University; Dr. Claude Fischler, director of research at the Centre national de la recherche scientifique (CNRS); Professor Michel de Lorgeril at the University of Grenoble and CNRS; Professor Declan Naughton at Kingston University; Dr. Annie Sasco, cancer epidemiologist at Bordeaux University; Dr. David Servan-Schreiber, author of *Anticancer, A New Way of Life*; Professor Stephen Taylor at the University of Queensland; Dr. Rachel Thompson at the World Cancer Research Fund for advising on my Anti-Cancer Challenge (www.zestforlifediet.com); Professor Carlo la Vecchia at the University of Milan; and Pierre Weill, agronomist and founder of *Bleu-Banc-Coeur*.

Words cannot even begin to express my deep and lasting gratitude to Glenn for his unflagging support during the two years it took me to write this book. He put up with a permanently disorganised home and wife and lent invaluable support as recipe critic, discussion partner, financial sponsor and fellow food-lover, helping me through difficult times and believing in this idea.

Last but not least, heartfelt thanks to our three wonderful children who munched their way through all these recipes, offering feedback, cheering me on and forgiving me for spending too much time in my study. This book is for the four of you.

Introduction

Eleven years ago I had a close brush with cancer. Diagnosed with cancerous lesions of the cervix, I decided to adopt a healthier lifestyle to support my medical treatment. However, I struggled to find reliable information and practical guidance to help me make the necessary changes.

There is more information available now than a decade ago but much of it is confusing and not based on solid medical science. Moreover, while many cancer-prevention books issue *theoretical* dietary recommendations, few provide guidance on *practical* ways of applying these in our busy day-to-day lives. This is why I decided to write this book.

My first aim is to help you rediscover the guilt-free pleasure of eating healthy, delicious food. Many of us worry about the potential health risks of what we eat. With respect to highly processed factory foods, such fears may be justified. However, when healthy eating feels like a grim duty or a joyless medical prescription, I do not believe that it can fulfill its true objective.

I say: Let's put pleasure back on the menu! When enjoying a varied diet of fresh, natural ingredients such as the one described in this book, don't be afraid of your food: savor it, have fun with it and celebrate it. It's the Mediterranean way.

Let's also put common sense back on the menu. Adding turmeric to every dish we eat, or consuming a pound of raw cabbage daily because we have heard that it may be beneficial, isn't common sense. If anything, we should avoid repetitive, one-dimensional diets; as we will see later, the healthiest diet is one that is rich in a *wide variety* of fresh, natural ingredients, carefully prepared and enjoyed with a positive and relaxed attitude.

Alas, nutritional common sense has become rare. If we followed the advice of our great-grandmothers ("eat your greens," "eat breakfast like a king, lunch like a nobleman, supper like a pauper," "chew your food properly" and "don't snack between meals") the western world would probably not be plagued with cancer, heart disease, diabetes and obesity.

So let's rediscover some of these ancient nourishing wisdoms: enjoying seasonal vegetables, putting a little more thought and time into what we consume, eating meals (rather than snacks) and enjoying these at dining tables instead of desks or cars, may just be some of the healthy habits worth rediscovering.

Tasty advice based on nutritional science

Zest for Life is a nutrition guide and cookbook in one. It aims to present the science of dietary cancer prevention *and* to show practical, enjoyable ways of integrating these findings into your daily life. It is the book I wanted when I was ill and that I am now making available to others wishing to prevent or overcome cancer.

Sadly, most of us have experienced cancer, either first-hand or because a loved one, friend or acquaintance has been afflicted by the disease. However, many cancers are preventable and what we eat (and don't eat) significantly affects our risk of developing the disease, as we will see later.

Chapters 2 to 4 discuss the link between food and cancer and the protective role of the Mediterranean diet. The research cited here is by no means definitive and further investigations are needed to shed more light on many unproven nutritional hypotheses.

Alas, human intervention studies, the types of research that could yield the most useful results in the area of dietary cancer-prevention, are difficult. Not only are they long and costly, such investigations also involve ethical dilemmas. For testing foods on humans to assess their potentially harmful effects (for instance, high intakes of processed meats, or soy in women at risk of breast cancer) might damage the health of the people being studied.

Uncertainty should not, however, prevent us from eating foods widely thought to have anti-cancer virtues, even if these have not been proven beyond doubt. Enjoying a wide variety of fresh, nourishing whole foods and avoiding nutrient-depleted, calorie-rich convenience products is likely to provide significant protection against cancer. Let's simply remember that there is no "miracle food" or nutrient that can prevent, let alone cure, cancer.

This book is not only for cancer patients. It is aimed more generally at those who wish to boost their defenses against a disease that has taken on epidemic proportions: worldwide, approximately a third of all people will get cancer at one point in their lives and one quarter will die of the disease[1].

Diet is not the only thing that affects our cancer risk. Among lifestyle factors that we can influence, regular physical activity is also crucial, as is maintaining a healthy body weight, avoiding tobacco and excess alcohol, carefully managing our exposure to sunlight and identifying and treating potentially cancer-causing infections[2]. Genes matter too, though less than people think: only about 5-10% of cancer cases are thought to be due to inherited genetic predispositions to cancer.

Environmental pollution and radiation are risk factors too, though unfortunately they are hard to avoid.

Since this book concerns itself primarily with nutrition and cooking we will leave these factors aside; for more information on various lifestyle cancer protection measures, see *Resources* (Appendix 5, p. 270).

The Mediterranean diet: delicious and nutritious

If you want to start cooking immediately, go straight to Chapter 5 (p. 97) which suggests many practical ways in which busy people can obtain, prepare and enjoy healthy foods every day. This is followed by more than 150 healthy anti-cancer recipes. They offer easy, delicious ways of eating the kinds of natural, fresh foods that our bodies thrive on.

The recipes in this book are grounded in the pre-industrial Mediterranean diet, a style of eating whose health benefits are supported by a vast body of research dating back to the 1950s[3]. It is rich in protective plant foods and omits the highly processed foods that characterize the typical western diet. As research is increasingly showing, the Mediterranean diet may offer protection not only from cancer but also from cardiovascular disease, diabetes, obesity and even depression and dementia.

Over and above merely biochemical considerations, the Mediterranean diet embodies freshness, diversity, simplicity, conviviality and *joie de vivre*. Healthy food should not feel like a punishment or a chore; if it does, we wouldn't eat that way for long.

Thankfully, the Mediterranean diet requires no sacrifices and tastes delicious, as the worldwide popularity of Italian and French food attests. This means that we can eat it indefinitely, as an enjoyable, healthy lifestyle habit rather than a prescriptive, restrictive "diet."

This book aims to show how life-affirming the Mediterranean way can be: shopping for seasonal ingredients, transforming them into tasty meals and savoring these consciously may in itself have therapeutic value, with positive ripple effects into other aspects of your life. This is why I have called the book *Zest for Life*: the title is not only a salute to one of my favorite anti-cancer ingredients, lemon zest, but also aims to awaken in readers feelings of energy, joyfulness and an appetite for life.

Controlling the controllables

Unfortunately, there is little we currently can do to reduce the cancer risks that may emanate from our genes, from environmental pollutants or from radiation. Therefore, we should do whatever we can to "control the controllables," that is, to make whatever healthy lifestyle changes *are* within our reach to help reduce our risk of developing cancer. This includes eating a healthy diet, regular physical activity, managing our stress levels and getting adequate sleep.

The highly respected World Cancer Research Fund Global Network (WCRF), an international not-for-profit organization that includes the American Institute for Cancer Research (AICR), has produced a list of 10 recommendations for cancer prevention (opposite)[4] based on an exhaustive analysis of the research into the link between diet and cancer which it published in its Expert Report in 2007.

Check the list and see how many you already practice. Next, decide which additional measures you want to adopt and integrate them, one by one, into your life. This book should help you get there.

Zest for Life supports cancer charities

I am donating a portion of the proceeds from the sale of this book to cancer charities (details regarding charitable donations can be found on the book's website: www. zestforlifediet.com).

I also wish to state that in writing this book I did not receive any support – direct or indirect – from food or pharmaceutical companies, supplement manufacturers or anyone else who might have a commercial interest in cancer treatment and/or prevention.

This is not to say that I have worked in isolation. Notably the WCRF has been assisting my blog, the Anti-Cancer Challenge (www.zestforlifediet.com), by providing expert advice, and much of this information has made its way into this book.

Moreover, to ensure that this book rests on solid scientific foundations, I have enlisted the advice of leading research scientists in the field of dietary cancer prevention and the Mediterranean diet. I am extremely grateful for their help; their work is cited throughout the book.

I have written this book using American spellings and terminology. For the avoidance of any misunderstandings, British and Australian terms are listed in a glossary at the back of the book, along with a metric/imperial conversion chart for measurements and temperatures. The recipes use *both* metric and imperial measurements.

WCRF/AICR recommendations for cancer prevention

1. Be as lean as possible without becoming underweight.

2. Be physically active for at least 30 minutes every day.

3. Limit consumption of energy-dense foods (foods that are high in fats and/or added sugars and/or low in fiber) and avoid sugary drinks.

4. Eat more of a variety of vegetables, fruits, whole grains and legumes, such as beans.

5. Limit consumption of red meats (such as beef, pork and lamb) and avoid processed meats.

6. If consumed at all, limit alcoholic drinks to two per day for men and one for women.

7. Limit consumption of salty foods and foods processed with salt (sodium).

8. Don't use supplements to protect against cancer.

9. It is best for mothers to breastfeed exclusively for up to six months and then to add other liquids and foods.

10. After treatment, cancer survivors should follow the recommendations for cancer prevention.

And, always remember – do not smoke or chew tobacco.

Chapter One

A Fresh Look at Food

When people think of cancer, they rarely associate it with food. However, it is increasingly understood that an anti-cancer diet can significantly lower our cancer risk.

According to the World Cancer Research Fund/American Institute for Cancer Research (WCRF/AICR), up to 30% of all cancers can be prevented by lifestyle and nutritional measures[1]. Others estimate that some of the commonest forms of cancer, such as breast, colorectal and prostate cancer, could be reduced by up to 70% and lung cancers by up to 50% if people ate an anti-cancer diet[2]. And in people who already have cancer, some studies suggest this type of diet may improve chances for recovery[3].

Nutrition is certainly not a stand-alone cancer treatment, nor is it a foolproof tool for prevention. Modern medical approaches are an essential part of any cancer therapy. Nonetheless, what and how you eat before, during and after cancer treatment may have a crucial impact on its outcome. And for people who are healthy but worry about becoming ill – without prevention, one in two men and one in three women living in the industrialized west will develop some form of cancer[4] – it's important to know that changes in diet can tip the odds in your favor.

Many hold the fatalistic belief that cancer is programmed by our genes and that there's nothing we can do about it. Even those who *are* aware that lifestyle plays a critical role in cancer usually think only of smoking, alcohol consumption or sun exposure as risk factors. Few consider food as something that can influence our cancer risk.

Once cancer has been diagnosed, most people embark on the recommended medical treatment: surgery, chemotherapy, radiation therapy, or a combination thereof. Most medical students are taught only the bare essentials of nutritional science and consequently, few doctors recommend dietary measures. Nevertheless, nutrition plays an important role in cancer prevention and recovery.

Healthy eating isn't just for cancer patients. There are benefits to everyone in a diet that boosts general health and well-being. The *Zest for Life* diet can potentially help prevent or relieve a long list of other medical conditions, including diabetes, cardiovascular disease, dementia, obesity and even depression.

Since the type of health-enhancing diet I propose in this book has no known negative side effects and may, in fact, have powerful benefits, we have every reason to adopt eating habits that may make the difference in preventing or overcoming cancer. Possible "side effects" will be increased energy, fewer colds, clearer skin and better digestion – something many people are happy to put up with!

Changing for good

Many of us know that we should eat plenty of fresh vegetables and fruit, whole grains, nuts and seeds, lean meat and oily fish and cut back on sugar, unhealthy fats or excess alcohol in order to look and feel better. However, few of us actually do it.

What's stopping us from making healthier choices? In most cases, there is a whole host of reasons: long-standing habits, time constraints, cost considerations and pressure from people around us, to name but a few.

Preparing healthy, home-made meals doesn't *have* to take much time. Most of the recipes in this book should take approximately 30-45 minutes to prepare, and even less if you can get help from a partner, children or friends. By organizing your food shopping and cooking and using some basic kitchen appliances, you can save a lot of time (see p. 106 for *Time saving tips.*).

Another reason we eat badly is cost. Aggressive marketing by producers of prepared foods and fast-food outlets has convinced many consumers that it costs less to eat convenience foods than to cook meals from scratch. Economic woes often reinforce the belief that healthy eating is an expensive luxury.

Not so! Many simple dishes – a salad of grated carrots or a batch of home-made tomato sauce – are much cheaper when cooked from scratch than bought ready-made. The use of fresh, basic ingredients means they will contain more nutrients and fewer unhealthy additives than their commercial equivalents. They will probably taste better, too.

While it is true that some convenience foods do carry a lower price tag than home-made meals, they also contain fewer nutrients. A considerable amount of the ingredients in convenience foods are fatty or starchy fillers with little nutritional value. With these products, you get what you pay for: their price may be low, but so is their nutritional value - and the cost in health terms can be considerable (see p. 108 for *Healthy eating on a budget.*).

Junk food advertising

There is one group of people who definitely would like us to continue eating unhealthy foods: their manufacturers and advertisers. A recent study[5] in the UK reported that over 25% of food advertisements in the most widely-read women's magazines were for ready-meals, sauces and soups high in salt and sugar.

A further 23% of the foods advertised had a high fat or sugar content, such as ice-cream, chocolate bars, candy and soft drinks. In contrast, only 1.8% of the advertisements were for fruits or vegetables.

Freeing ourselves from these harmful messages is one more step towards a healthy diet. The best way to do this is to buy only fresh food in its natural state, food that has undergone as little processing (refining, baking, cooking, packaging or preserving) as possible. Wherever possible, we should try to buy seasonal, locally-grown foods directly from their producers.

Another widespread reason for poor eating habits is that they are, well, habits, deeply ingrained. Habits are a largely unreflective way of doing things because that is the way we, and often our parents before us, have always done them. To break a habit, we must first become aware of it. Only then can we ask ourselves, "Is this habit serving me well? Is it making me fit and healthy, and protecting my body from disease?" If the answer is "no," it's time to let go of it.

It is not always easy to spot which habits are making us unwell. Indeed, often we don't even realize we *are* unwell, as many of us have forgotten what it feels like to be truly fit and healthy. Poor health has crept up on us over the years and we assume it is simply related to ageing. In many cases, however, our health has deteriorated not as a result of age, but of lifestyle.

Meanwhile, many poor eating habits are hard to shake off because they are deeply rooted in our emotions. Some foods, especially those high in sugar and fat, make us feel good quickly and so we seek them out.

The first flavor we experience in infancy is the sweet taste of milk. We learn to associate it with comfort, security and love. During childhood, we are offered sweet treats to cheer us up when we are sad, to reward us for being brave at a difficult time, or for being good when our parents need us to be. Thus, sugary food becomes a reward, an incentive or a token of love and is inextricably woven into our emotional fabric.

As adults we are free to indulge in unhealthy feel-good treats at every turn: when we are having a good day (reward), a bad one (comfort), when we feel self-indulgent (a well-deserved luxury) or underprivileged (a rare treat). Many of us use sugar to boost flagging energy levels, a message reinforced by the food industry's enthusiastic claims about the "energizing" qualities of sugar.

Because they make us feel so good, we get emotionally and biochemically hooked on some foods – especially sweet, starchy or caffeinated ones. Such habits are hard to break, but defensive strategies can help us override these urges and adopt new, healthier eating patterns. This book offers practical suggestions to help you break away from habits that do not serve you well.

External pressures against change

Sometimes the people around us act as an obstacle to dietary change. Spouses, children, parents or friends may – consciously or unconsciously – sabotage our efforts to change our diet. In some cases, they may feel challenged by our new way of eating as it calls their own dietary choices into question.

Spouses may mutter darkly about red meat or sugar deprivation; children may complain at having to eat more vegetables. Parents – especially mothers – may feel offended because we are rejecting food they have prepared for us. ("But you've always *loved* my caramel fudge cake!") Colleagues or friends may ridicule our new "fad" diet and predict we won't be able to stay the course.

Faced with these challenges, we need to gather up all the strength and confidence we can muster and tell ourselves, "I am doing this for myself. I know my body's needs better than anyone and this is what I need to eat in order to stay healthy."

Do not try to force your family or friends into adopting your way of eating. All you can do is to tell them calmly that you want to eat differently and that this is important to you. Start by cooking some of the recipes in this book. Once they realize how committed you are, how much better you feel as a result of your dietary changes and how delicious your meals look, smell and taste, they may eventually join you.

Cook for yourself

Many of us don't know how to cook — another factor preventing us from adopting a healthier diet.

One way to learn may be to attend cookery classes. A simpler option is proposed in this book: recipes that require little more than basic kitchen equipment, some inexpensive ingredients and enthusiasm to experiment and learn.

If you are new to cooking, begin with the easiest recipes and build on these as your culinary confidence increases. Some people like to acquire new skills in company: you could ask a few friends, colleagues or family members to meet up regularly for a "Healthy Cooking Club" which could provide a convivial experience of preparing food together and sharing it afterwards in a relaxed setting.

Start by closely sticking to the recipes in this book. As you become more confident, feel free to substitute ingredients as you like and eventually, to develop new recipes loosely based on the ones you first prepared. When you taste the result of your labors, you can be justifiably flushed with pride at the fact that you made a meal from scratch, with your own hands and imagination.

Cooking doesn't have to be a chore

Cooking your own food can provide a wonderfully creative outlet. Many of us feel we have little space in our lives for true creativity; the kitchen is a place where you can really let your creative juices flow. Cooking is also a very effective way to unwind, provided you don't impose performance or time pressure on yourself.

Preparing simple, quick dishes after a long day can be surprisingly relaxing: hearing the rhythmic chopping sounds of the knife on the wooden board, inhaling the invigorating aroma of freshly crushed garlic or the comforting smell of warm olive oil, marveling at the vibrant colors of red bell peppers, bright green zucchini or glistening purple eggplant, or licking a drop of lemony vinaigrette off your fingertip can crowd out your noisy thoughts for just a few moments and let your other senses — smell, touch, taste, sight — take over.

Make changes one meal at a time

Dietary change doesn't happen overnight; it is an ongoing journey, and with time you will get better at it. Some people get frustrated by the difficulty of making significant changes in their diet and give up before their new habits have yielded tangible results.

To avoid this happening, be kind to yourself and give yourself time. You don't have to "get it right" straight away. As long as you keep working to improve your diet, even in small steps, you are reducing your risks of developing cancer and improving your chances for overall health.

The first step is to *add* new, healthy foods and drinks to your existing diet. Once you are happy eating and drinking these, the next step – *removing unhealthy foods* – will come much more easily.

For example: if you regularly eat frozen fish sticks with instant mashed potatoes, you can begin by adding a serving of broccoli to this meal. Next, you could replace the mashed potatoes with home-made Pumpkin mash (p. 221) or Cauliflower mash (p. 218). Then, you could swap the packaged fish sticks for one of the tasty fresh fish dishes in this book (p. 164-176). Before you know it, you've vastly improved the quality of your diet *and* broadened your culinary repertoire!

This type of gradual dietary shift – which can take place over several weeks, months or years – will help prevent a sense of shock or deprivation, making your dietary changes more sustainable in the long run.

Eating fresh, natural foods – ideally in a relaxed environment, with people whose company you enjoy – can set in motion a powerful positive cycle. For instance, healthier food may help us feel more energetic. Feeling more energetic will encourage us to exercise more. Physical activity coupled with healthy, fresh food may improve the quality of our sleep. All three together may help bring about a more positive outlook on life. Thus, taking control of our health can have powerful benefits, not just physical but also emotional!

My journey towards health

In writing this book I wanted to share the insights and experiences that have helped me return to a more healthful, balanced way of eating. As I improved my diet over the years, other aspects of my life were transformed as well. Not only have I been able to resist serious disease, I have also come to enjoy high levels of energy, resilience and creativity I had not known before.

My nutritional learning curve has been characterized by a pattern of "two steps forward, one step back." I don't pretend to be a paragon of nutritional virtue and understand the difficulties inherent in making significant dietary changes. However, I hope this book can help you to avoid some of the pitfalls I experienced and to discover the rewards of the healthy, energizing diet I propose here. My journey of nutritional discovery continues to this day; I invite you to join me.

Re-learning to eat

Luckily for me, my mother learned to cook the old-fashioned way. She would boil up cauldrons of nourishing broths containing great hunks of marrow bone, aromatic herbs and vegetables; she prepared home-made jams and spicy fruit compotes, and steered well clear of preserved and prepackaged foods. Operating on a tight budget, my mother bought seasonal produce directly from local growers. In the main, I enjoyed a healthy diet; however, candy, home-made cakes and refined breakfast cereals also featured regularly, as did smoked sausages and ham.

From the age of 18 months I suffered severe eczema that covered most of my body; no doctor was able to find an explanation for my skin affliction, and the only solution provided was cortisone cream. I later came to realize that it might have been caused by an allergy to cow's milk.

As I grew older, I also began suffering a wide range of embarrassing digestive complaints, chronic sinusitis, debilitating bouts of fatigue and constant yeast infections. Looking back, I don't remember ever feeling fully healthy during my youth and early adult years. Knowing nothing about natural medicine and having been declared "incurable," I assumed I would simply have to suffer a lifetime of itching, bloating and sniffling.

Some 10 years later, intense stress levels compounded my already fragile health. I was living in central London, working in a stressful job as a journalist at the *Financial Times* and feeling exhausted all the time. My diet was a disaster: when I wasn't skipping breakfast altogether, it was a sugar-laden pastry or a bagel washed down with coffee in a polystyrene cup on the train to work.

Lunch most days was a packaged sandwich. I snacked regularly on cookies or potato chips and drank coffee throughout the day. Dinner was often pasta with ready-made sauce, or Indian or Chinese take-out. Vegetables made rare, almost accidental appearances and my busy schedule made shopping and cooking difficult.

Over the years, I consulted many specialists for my many health problems — not only orthodox medical specialists, but also homeopaths, herbalists, acupuncturists and even a faith healer. None were able to help.

One day, on a reporting assignment, I was interviewing a doctor near my office about the health effects of chronic stress. As he talked to me about the nutritional factors affecting health, it dawned on me that nutritional changes might help me. At a subsequent consultation, he recommended I cut out milk, wheat, yeast and sugar for three months, drastically increase my intake of vegetables and drink less coffee. Imagine my horror upon hearing that I would have to replace 80% of my diet!

Changing my eating habits was a struggle, but soon I began to feel better than I had in years. My energy levels climbed, I lost excess weight, my skin and sinuses cleared up and I felt healthier and happier than I had for a long time. I was so inspired by the improvements I was experiencing that I decided to leave journalism and begin a four-year training course to become a nutritional therapist.

A few years later, at 33, I was eating a healthier – though by no means ideal – diet and my stress levels remained sky-high as I juggled caring for my three year-old son, my marriage, nutrition studies and part-time journalism work. One sunny June morning, my gynecologist called me at work and I could tell by his voice that something wasn't right. My Pap smear had shown severe cellular abnormalities; a follow-up test revealed *carcinoma in situ* – cancerous lesions of the cervix.

I was extremely lucky: the cancer cells hadn't spread. They were surgically removed and I was spared the traumatic treatment I might have had to undergo had I been diagnosed a few months later. But the shock of the diagnosis was my wake-up call, and I decided to make significant changes. While my illness had been primarily caused by infection by the human papilloma virus (HPV), my sub-optimal diet and high-stress lifestyle had encouraged the disease to unfold. And so I finally began eating as though my life depended on it.

Dietary overhaul

It has taken me years, but I have now fundamentally changed my diet. I have developed a love for vegetables and fruit, which I now eat for pleasure rather than because I feel I have to. I have cut right back on sugary foods and refined starch. I eat small amounts of meat, mostly poultry, and I regularly consume oily fish. Cows' milk has been largely replaced by nut beverages and cows' cheese by goats' and ewes' milk cheeses.

Living in the countryside, with its year-round supply of delicious and nutritious food has made healthy eating easier. I buy most of my vegetables from a farmer in my village or at a farmers' market, and we grow some vegetables in a small kitchen garden. Meat comes from local organic farms, health food shops or a local butcher who sells traditionally reared meat. In our garden, six chickens roam, eating slugs, snails and worms and occasional grains. They lay the tastiest eggs I have ever eaten.

I am reaping the benefits of my lifestyle changes. My skin and sinus problems have gone, my energy levels are high, I rarely catch a cold more than once a year, my digestive system works smoothly and my Pap smears have kept coming in clear.

Ongoing lifestyle changes

I can't pretend to be a nutritional saint. At certain times – especially when I'm feeling stressed or tired – I crave sugary or starchy comfort foods (bread for instance), and if I have them in reach, I find it hard to hold back. I usually pay the price for my transgression within hours, in the form of sinus congestion, abdominal bloating and fatigue. So over the years I've developed strategies to protect me from myself.

The most effective measure is simply not to stock overly tempting foods in my house. Candy, cookies and potato chips were banished years ago; more recently, I also started keeping only a small supply of bread on hand (I freeze the rest, pre-sliced for easy defrosting). The chocolate I buy is so intense (80-95% cocoa content) that I cannot eat more than one or two squares at a time.

I stock tasty, healthy foods in my house, car and handbag, so that when I feel an urge to snack, I am forced to dip into the fruit bowl or eat a few nuts – surprisingly satisfying when there's nothing else available! I also make sure to eat regular, balanced meals to avoid feeling ravenous at mealtimes or craving unhealthy snacks in-between.

Another major shift occurred in my early 30s when I started to cook regularly. My first culinary attempts during my student days were such a disaster that I'd abandoned the whole idea. However, once I became a mother I realized that I was now responsible for feeding not just myself but also a fast-growing child with important nutritional needs, and so I started to cook.

My cooking career progressed in fits and starts, with quite a few mishaps along the way. (The most notorious of these was a gigantic potato that I'd left to boil unattended for hours and that was eventually reduced to a small chunk of charcoal while I was off doing other things. My family still teases me about this.)

I bought a few cookbooks and started experimenting in the kitchen, and my confidence soon began to grow. My life-long love of tasty food, coupled with a dislike of eating the same things repeatedly, spurred me on to try out new dishes and ingredients.

The internet has been a gold mine of information, offering answers regarding novel foods and leading me into new directions. It also provides a great forum for sharing ideas and recipes with other people who have similar health concerns.

Another healthy-eating tactic I have developed over the years – I call it "substitutionism" – allows me to eat foods that *taste like* sweet, fatty junk but are actually very healthy. I do this by replacing ingredients like butter, sugar or white flour with healthier alternatives such as olive oil, acacia honey and ground almonds. These allow me to fool my body into thinking that it just got a quick sugar hit when in fact I have eaten a nutrient-dense snack that will keep me going for hours.

On long car or airplane journeys, I bring along a nutritional survival kit to avoid eating poor-quality snacks and sandwiches. It includes a stainless-steel tub with nuts, seeds and dried fruit, a hard-boiled egg, bruise-resistant fresh fruit (apples and oranges) or home-made sandwiches prepared with wholegrain bread and healthy fillings like *Sardinade* (p. 122). This isn't only tasty and healthy, but a lot cheaper than processed airport and roadside snacks.

My friends and family have been supportive of my evolving dietary habits. My husband, himself passionate about healthy food, enthusiastically encourages my culinary experiments. Our children rarely grumble about having to eat healthy food and seem to enjoy most of the meals I prepare. Amazingly, considering my humble beginnings, I now teach healthy-cooking classes to people who want to improve their diets but don't know how to cook.

Over the years I have learned to listen to my body and to interpret its signals. I am now able to distinguish fatigue induced by a low blood-sugar level (leaden, mind-numbing and overpowering) from "good old-fashioned" fatigue caused by a busy day or lack of sleep (burning eyes, yawning). I can tell when my desire to eat is prompted by real hunger (a gnawing sensation at the pit of my stomach), or by boredom or frustration (obsessive thoughts about chocolate and bread).

After many years of ignoring it, getting to know my body didn't happen overnight. It took a lot of patient, careful listening and a process of trial and error to find out what worked and what didn't. Over time, I have learned that recognizing and meeting my body's needs for the right food, exercise and rest has gone hand in hand with a growing sense of self-awareness and, dare I say: self-love.

Seen in this light, healthy nutrition can be about much more than mere nourishment; it is a way of nurturing the very core of one's being, comforting it and giving it what it needs.

Chapter Two

The Mediterranean Diet

When I began writing this book I analyzed the eating habits I had adopted over the years – rich in vegetables, fruits, whole grains and nuts, high in olive oil and fatty fish, relatively low in red meat or dairy – and it struck me: without consciously intending to do so, I had adopted the traditional Mediterranean diet.

The term "Mediterranean diet" has become a fashionable buzzword; yet, this way of eating has been around for thousands of years. Unlike many modern health-food regimes, the Mediterranean style of eating was not deliberately designed as a way to boost human health and longevity. Nor should it be seen as a time-limited "diet" for weight-loss. Rather, the Mediterranean diet is simply a traditional way of eating that evolved naturally, organically, in response to climatic and ecological conditions.

The many different soils and micro-climates found in various parts of the Mediterranean basin have produced a high degree of variation among foods and flavors across the region. As a result, each area has its celebrated specialties: for example, herbs, olive oil and summer vegetables from Provence in southern France; ewes' milk cheese and olives from Greece; durum wheat or parmesan from Italy; garlic, beans and almonds from Spain; pungent herbs and spices, beans and garbanzos and a profusion of fresh and dried fruits from North Africa and the Middle East – to name only a few.

Despite this wide diversity of flavors, ingredients and preparation methods, the region's traditional food patterns share many common traits. Because natural conditions were not particularly conducive to intensive animal husbandry, the inhabitants of the Mediterranean basin traditionally ate an abundance of plant foods: vegetables and fruits, weeds, roots and berries, nuts and seeds foraged in the wild, beans and legumes.

Grains were consumed in their natural, unrefined state, mostly in the form of bread baked from whole, coarse barley or spelt flour, using sourdough as leavening, or as gruels cooked with water. Sugar was largely absent, processed food non-existent.

A profusion of plant foods

To this day, plant foods remain at the heart of the Mediterranean cuisine. Take a look at any Greek, Spanish, Lebanese or Italian restaurant menu. Here you can choose between salads of roasted bell peppers, onions and eggplant sprinkled with fresh herbs, or an *antipasto* of artichoke hearts marinated in olive oil.

There may be Marinated mushrooms (p. 123), chilled Gazpacho (p. 152), Hummus (p. 192) or crunchy Garbanzo falafels nestling on a bed of crisp lettuce and doused with garlicky sesame sauce (p. 190). For dessert, succulent figs stewed in red wine, baked peaches or, more simply, mixed nuts and dried fruits are on offer.

With its heavy emphasis on plant foods, the pre-industrial Mediterranean diet was virtually vegetarian. This was reinforced by religious practices that dominated the region's eating habits until only two or three decades ago.

Especially the Eastern Orthodox, Catholic and Armenian Churches limited or restricted meat: all animal foods – sometimes even eggs and dairy – were prohibited for forty days before Christmas and 10 days afterwards, the 40 days leading up to Easter, the 15 days before the Feast of the Assumption on August 15, as well as on every Wednesday and Friday of the year.

What modest amounts of animal protein were eaten came mainly from wild fish caught in the sea, rivers and lakes; from meager yields of goats' or ewes' milk used to make yogurt or cheese; from the eggs and flesh of chickens scratching around the yard, and from occasional goat meat, wild rabbits and game birds, such as geese, ducks, pheasant or quail, whose lean, aromatic flesh provided flavor to vegetable stews and soups. Wild, foraged animal foods like snails and frogs, an excellent source of healthy fats and protein, remain popular in France to this day.

Pulling all these tasty and healthy ingredients together, olive oil has been the principal source of fat around the Mediterranean for thousands of years, prized for its rich flavor and high nutritional value. Further stimulating its eaters' taste buds, the region's diet has always made copious use of pungent garlic, aromatic herbs – oregano, thyme, parsley or fresh cilantro – and spices such as turmeric, ginger, cumin and coriander.

You too can eat like a Mediterranean

You may be wondering how you can adopt a Mediterranean diet without moving to Greece or Italy (albeit perhaps a tempting thought). The good news is: you can eat this way wherever you live!

The Mediterranean diet: top-10 Features

1. High intake of **vegetables and fruits**

2. High intake of **olive oil**

3. High intake of **legumes (pulses), whole grains, nuts and seeds**

4. Frequent use of **aromatic herbs and spices**

5. Moderate-to-high intake of **fish and eggs**

6. Moderate consumption of **dairy products**, mostly as cheese and yogurt

7. Moderate intake of **meat** and meat products

8. Moderate **wine** consumption with meals (where accepted by religion)

9. Absence of mass-produced **processed food**; low intake of sugar, refined flour products and industrially refined fats

10. Central role of **conviviality**: sharing food and drink with others

Based on ingredients that are easily available everywhere, simple to prepare and delicious, Mediterranean-style eating can be transported to any part of the globe and adapted to local conditions (seasons, types of vegetables and fruits grown there). Indeed, many adherents of the Mediterranean diet living in northern Europe, the U.S. or Australia are reaping its benefits daily[1-3].

Sadly, one of the most reliable indicators of the healthiness of the Mediterranean diet is that when populations give up this style of eating, their health deteriorates markedly. Many citizens of modern-day Greece, Spain and Italy no longer eat the traditional Mediterranean diet, having replaced it with lower-quality fast food, and they're paying the price in terms of declining health, notably through a sharp increase in obesity.

The optimal cancer-prevention diet

Over the millennia, the wide diversity in foods and flavors around the Mediterranean gave rise to markedly distinct and diverging culinary traditions. But what is striking is that almost *every* food thought to have anti-cancer properties – such as garlic, onions, cabbage, berries, green tea, mushrooms, olive oil, oily fish, nuts, seeds, lentils, aromatic herbs, spices and a wide and colorful range of fruit and vegetables – is an integral part of the traditional Mediterranean diet, no matter which region.

From a purely biological perspective, in terms of the range and depth of nutrients it supplies, the pre-industrial Mediterranean diet is probably the closest thing to the optimal anti-cancer diet.

It is unclear whether the Mediterranean diet actually prevents the formation of tumors or whether its protective role lies in hindering micro-tumors from developing into full-blown, life-threatening cancer. Whatever the mechanism, scientists estimate that up to 25% of colorectal cancers, 15% of breast cancers and 10% of prostate, pancreas, and endometrial cancers could be prevented if people living in the industrialized west did nothing more than adopt a Mediterranean diet[4].

The more closely people adhere to the Mediterranean diet, the greater its anti-cancer effect is thought to be. According to a study conducted in Greece during the late 1990s, strict adherence to two elements of the Mediterranean diet – for example, a high consumption of vegetables and a low intake of meat – was found to bring about a 12% reduction in the incidence of all cancers[5]. The more elements of the Mediterranean diet were incorporated, the greater their protection; thus, adhering to four elements – for instance, by adding a high intake of fruits and legumes to the two measures described above – might reduce cancer incidence by up to 24%.

When combined with other healthy lifestyle habits, the Mediterranean style of eating may confer *even* greater protection. A large-scale European study conducted over 12 years showed that people eating a Mediterranean diet who hadn't smoked for 15 years or longer, undertook regular physical activity and drank a moderate amount of alcohol were 65% more likely to outlive those who had none of these healthy habits and were 60% less likely to die of cancer[6].

The only controlled dietary investigation to date into the health effects of the Mediterranean diet yielded similar results. The Lyon Diet Heart Study[7] indicated that eating a Mediterranean diet not only protected its 605 participants from cardiovascular disease, but also from cancer.

Patients in the experimental group were encouraged to follow a regimen rich in fruits, vegetables and whole grains, to replace some meat with fish, to use healthy oils (especially omega-3 fats, see Chapter 3) and avoid unhealthy fats, and were allowed to drink moderate amounts of red wine with meals. After four years, they were found to be 61% less likely to develop cancer than members of the control group they were being compared to and who were eating the American Heart Association's so-called prudent diet!

Is there a "secret ingredient"?

For decades, scientists have debated passionately about what exactly it is about the Mediterranean diet that makes it so healthy. Is it the red wine? The olive oil? The high intake of vegetables? Garlic? Tomatoes or oily fish?

One important protective factor of the Mediterranean diet is its high proportion of vegetables, fruits and legumes. In addition to vitamins, minerals and fiber, these plant foods contain bioactive substances called phyto-chemicals ("phyto" is the ancient Greek word for "plant") thought to protect us from a wide range of diseases, including cancer. While scientific evidence for the protective effects of vegetables and fruits is mixed – some studies show greater protection than others – a diet rich in unprocessed plant foods may well cut cancer risks, if only by crowding out the less-healthy foods we might otherwise eat.

Vegetable and fruit consumption in many Mediterranean countries is higher than in many other western countries. Greeks eat up to 1¼ pounds (550 grams) of vegetables and 12 ounces (335 grams) of fruit each day[8]. The vegetables most commonly eaten in Greece include lettuce, cabbage, wild greens, tomatoes, green beans, eggplant, artichokes, cucumber, onions, garlic and legumes (such as lentils, beans and garbanzos). Citrus fruits, apples, pears, peaches, melon, watermelon and cherries are among the most widely consumed fruits.

By comparison, the average American eats 7¾ ounces (220 grams) of vegetables and 6 ounces (165 grams) of fruit each day[9]. Potatoes (which are not actually vegetables, but starchy tubers) make up for 27% of U.S. "vegetable" consumption. Meanwhile, bananas, and oranges and apples in the form of juice are the most popular fruits in the US. Cultivated to be particularly sweet, none of these three fruits can be considered anti-cancer foods, especially once they have been processed into juice.

Olive oil is thought to be another protective factor in the Mediterranean diet. Extra-virgin cold-pressed olive oil contains compounds called antioxidants that are thought to protect the body's cells against cancer-causing agents (free radicals) and its stable chemical structure makes it suitable for cooking at moderate temperatures.

The moderate meat intake characterizing the traditional Mediterranean diet may be another cancer-protective factor. Frequently eating red, processed or preserved meat is linked to cancer – especially colorectal, but also esophageal, lung, endometrial, stomach and pancreatic cancer[10,11]. Conversely, eating fish – a popular source of protein in places like Spain, Italy and North Africa – may confer added protection[12]. This is true especially of fish rich in omega-3 fatty acids, such as sardines, herring, mackerel and anchovies.

A large European study recently found that people eating as little as three ounces (80 grams) of fish daily – just over half a typical tin of sardines – cut their colon cancer risk by 30% compared to those eating little or none. Meanwhile a regular intake of red and processed meats pointed to increased risks: those eating more than 5½ ounces (160 grams) daily had a 35% higher risk of colon cancer than those eating less than one ounce (20 grams)[13].

Variety really is the spice of life: food synergy

While many individual foods traditionally consumed around the Mediterranean may have important cancer-protective characteristics, the benefits of the Mediterranean way of eating go well beyond the sum of its parts. It is the *combination* of these foods and their mutually reinforcing interaction that makes this diet so healthy. Scientists refer to this type of interaction as "food synergy," where one food reinforces the effects of another, providing greater health protection than if both foods were eaten separately.

In the past, much nutritional research focused on the effect of individual food components – for example protein, fiber, or vitamin C – on human health. But isolated compounds studied under laboratory conditions do not behave the same way they do when obtained from whole foods, or when they are eaten in combination with each other.

Many studies, for instance, have failed to show the health effects of fiber- or beta-carotene supplements (indeed, some have found increased cancer risk in smokers taking beta-carotene supplements). This doesn't mean that fiber or beta-carotene aren't important for health, but rather, that they are most effective when consumed in combination with other nutrients, and as whole foods.

Thus, the benefits of the Mediterranean diet may lie not so much in the individual foods that constitute it, but in the fact that they are eaten *together*, in a wide variety of combinations and preparations: some raw, others cooked; some dried, some fermented, others marinated in olive oil or lemon juice; some grated, others whole; at different stages of ripeness and varying times of the day.

Several studies have shown that eating a wide variety of healthy foods can protect us from a whole host of cancers, notably those of the digestive tract, from the mouth to the rectum[14-16], and from breast cancer[17]. The health effect of a varied diet is most noticeable with vegetables and fruits; varying different types of meat or cereal grains does not appear to have noticeable benefits. (We will return to food synergy in Chapter 4.)

Beyond molecules: a Mediterranean food culture

So far, we have discussed only the biological factors that make the Mediterranean diet so healthy. However, over and above the foods that make up this diet, the region boasts a unique eating culture: it's not just *what* people eat, but also *how* they eat that distinguishes the Mediterranean way of eating from other food cultures.

Regardless of regional differences and still relatively untouched by recent changes in eating habits, there remains an overarching Mediterranean food culture characterized by three key elements: variety, quality and conviviality.

Variety, Quality & Conviviality: The Mediterranean Diet's "Holy Trinity"

Variety *A wide range of foods can be found on French, Italian or Spanish dinner tables, where a traditional meal might include vegetable soup or meat broth as an appetizer followed by a mixed salad or a small portion of pasta, meat or fish and vegetables and rounded off by cheese or fruit. Each dish is modest in size but offers a vast array of nutrients.*

Quality *The first thing you notice when visiting a French or Italian market is how discerning shoppers are when it comes to selecting their purchases. Limp lettuce, over-ripe apricots or less-than-perfectly matured cheese will be cast aside. Shoppers do not hesitate to ask about the way the food was grown or to return purchases that were not up to their exacting standards. This insistence on quality ensures that the food on offer provides optimal nutrition and flavor.*

Conviviality *The most life-affirming aspect of Mediterranean food culture is the central role of conviviality, the pleasure of sharing food with others and of celebrating communal culinary traditions and life at large. Without it, the Mediterranean diet would be just another biological health-food prescription; conviviality, at its heart, makes it a way of life.*

Conviviality, the missing link

The word "convivial" comes from Latin, where it refers quite simply to the act of living together. We are drawn to conviviality by our human nature, our need for safety, companionship and comfort.

Conviviality need not involve expensive ingredients or complicated preparations; the simplest village *fête* can be an occasion of unbridled revelry in food that is jointly prepared and eaten. France, for one, boasts countless gastronomic festivals at which villages or entire regions celebrate their local agricultural product, sometimes over several days.

In Provence, the famous black Nyons olive is celebrated every January at a two-day event in the small town of Buis les Baronnies. The festival features a church blessing of the year's new oil crop, oil-tasting sessions, workshops teaching how to make *tapenade* (see p. 122 for recipe), an *aioli* taste-off (*aioli* is a garlic mayonnaise; see recipe on p. 166-7) and much gaiety around the olive-pit spitting competition.

On the Mediterranean coast near Marseilles, the fishing town of Martigues celebrates its seafood bounty every summer with so-called *sardinades,* events at which people grill and eat fresh sardines along the banks of the picturesque town's canals.

In the south-west of France, the garlic-growing town of Cadours holds a three-day festival every August to celebrate its unique purple garlic. The event features garlic-peeling demonstrations, artfully woven garlic sculptures and the sale of home-preserved garlic in olive oil. Past festivals have featured raucous clove-spitting contests and the selection of a garlic queen – crowned, of course, with a wreath of garlic!

The culinary high point of the Cadours garlic festival is the *tourin à l'ail* (see recipe on p. 145), a 40 gallon (150-litre) cauldron of garlic soup that is served – free of charge – to anyone who remembered to bring a soup bowl and spoon from home (and those who didn't are given disposable tableware – no one is allowed to leave with an empty stomach). In the balmy evening air infused with the scent of garlic, strangers come together around trestle tables under the 200-year-old red-brick market hall, getting acquainted and sharing a laugh as they savor a simple meal of garlic soup, crusty bread and a glass of the local red.

This celebration of the senses and the grateful, guilt-free acceptance of pleasure are typical of a Mediterranean meal. Taking time to prepare and savor our food consciously, without distraction or guilt, and, if possible, enjoying it with friends or loved ones, is one of the best things we can do for our health, both at a physical and an emotional level.

When snacking replaces meals

You don't need to leave your house or spend a lot of money to enjoy a moment of conviviality. All it takes is one person or more, a table, some chairs (even a picnic blanket will do) and some simple, tasty food.

While this may seem like the obvious definition of a standard meal, the sad fact is that more and more people snack their way through the day and eat fewer and fewer sit-down meals. Even if you are on your own, sitting down to eat in a pleasant place (not in front of the TV or the computer) will encourage healthy eating and conviviality with yourself.

A U.S. study found that among 18- to 50-year old Americans, roughly 20% of all meals are eaten in the car[18]. According to the U.S. National Highway Traffic Safety Administration, in-car eating is a more dangerous distraction than using a hand-held mobile phone while driving. Consequently, U.S. insurer Hagerty Classic compiled a list of the 10 most dangerous foods to eat while driving: chocolate came in first place (a distraction as drivers wipe their sticky fingers), followed by spill-prone drinks, squirty jam- or cream-filled donuts and greasy fried chicken.[19]

Meanwhile in Britain, a growing number of meals are eaten in front of the TV, in the car or standing around the kitchen; only 37% of families eat most of their meals at a dinner table, according to one survey[20]. Some 12% of respondents said they hardly ever eat with their family, and another 12% said they rarely speak during family mealtimes. One packaged gravy manufacturer even launched an advertising campaign to encourage British families to aspire to have one "proper" home-cooked meal together – per week!

When they do eat a meal, most people rush through it. The average British meal is eaten in just 14 minutes and 27 seconds, less than half the more leisurely 33 minutes spent chewing and chatting 20 years ago. Of the people surveyed, eight in 10 said they regularly snack in front of the television, with one in five eating in front of a computer. Meals are also gobbled down while reading, sending text messages or talking on the phone, and fewer than two in 10 respondents said they regularly give their plates their full attention. Some 73% of Britons don't bother using a knife at mealtimes and 64% eat food straight out of its packaging.

In today's hyper-efficient, fast-paced world, we often sacrifice that which made us human and which built our society: our fundamental need for food and the communality that was born of this need. This modern way of eating cannot provide humans with the biological or emotional sustenance they thrive on. I want to encourage you to rediscover the joys of eating calmly, at a table, using cutlery, ideally in the company of people you feel comfortable with.

Shared, leisurely meals are about much more than fueling our bodies, they are "uniquely human institutions where our species developed language and this thing we call culture," U.S. health writer Michael Pollan argues in an impassioned plea for a return to more traditional eating habits[21]. "The shared meal elevates eating from a mechanical process of fueling our body to a ritual of family and community, from mere animal biology to an act of culture."

Adopting a Mediterranean approach to eating

In recommending the Mediterranean diet, therefore, I want to move beyond the "food-as-medicine" paradigm, where food is seen merely as an amalgamation of molecules that support bodily functions and promote physical health (a mechanistic view popular in Anglo-Saxon countries).

Instead, I espouse the more holistic ethos prevalent in Mediterranean cultures where food is also a source of spiritual nourishment, of pleasure, comfort and vitality – a celebration of life in the fullest sense.

Although unhealthy modern eating patterns have been making inroads into Mediterranean countries, many retain a rich and joyful food culture. Indeed, French or Spanish restaurants at lunchtime throng with office workers enjoying a leisurely meal and engaged in lively conversations rarely pertaining to work. On Sundays, three-generation families gather around many a dining table for two to three hours' eating, relaxing and laughter. These groups often include babies and toddlers who learn from an early age that eating with others is an occasion for joy and communality.

Sociologists have compared habits of conviviality in Mediterranean and Anglo-Saxon countries and their results make fascinating reading. In an international survey of people's attitudes to food and eating, respondents were asked to describe what, to them, constituted a "healthy diet"[22].

Whereas primary health concerns for the Americans and Britons surveyed touched on notions such as "proteins," "carbohydrates" and "fat," Italian and French respondents overwhelmingly focused on the concept of pleasure. Indeed, during focus-group discussions, French participants mentioned the words "pleasure" and "joy" 79 times, whereas these terms came up only 16 times in the American group.

There was also a great divergence in respondents' attitudes to conviviality: when asked what constitutes a healthy diet, French and French-speaking Swiss participants spoke spontaneously of "family meals" or "eating with friends." In the French-speaking focus group, the word "family" came up 39 times, "friends" 51 times, "convivial" 72 times and "sharing" 38 times.

This is in striking contrast with the Anglophone groups, where "family" was mentioned eight times, "friends" four times and "sharing" only three times. Lastly, while Anglophones and Germans valued "conviviality" on special occasions, the French, in particular, said they treasured conviviality as an ordinary, day-to-day event.

In addition to their attachment to conviviality, the French and Italian respondents also adhered most closely to a strict set of rules about meal times (three meals a day, at fixed hours), portion sizes (modest), table manners (no phones, no TV), snacking between meals (forbidden), second helpings (frowned upon), dietary variety (essential), eating environments (tables, real dishes and cutlery, not cars, sidewalks or desks).

Thus, "Mediterranean" anti-cancer eating isn't just about eating healthy food. It's also about consciously developing a *health-promoting attitude to food.*

In recommending to you the Mediterranean diet, therefore, I refer also to its underlying philosophy, not just to specific anti-cancer ingredients. I am talking about fresh, natural food grown nearby in living earth, under open skies, moistened by rain, ripened by the sun and brimming with essential nutrients, simply prepared and enjoyed in a relaxed mood.

Indeed, this is very much in keeping with the spirit of Mediterranean culinary traditions, where dishes were rarely cooked in accordance with rigid rules and recipes, but rather, came together in an instinctive, organic way based on whatever ingredients were available and on the cook's ingenious ability to transform these into a simple yet tasty dish. Mediterranean cuisine is essentially an "anti-recipe"-cuisine; thus, the recipes in this book are meant less as rules to be adhered to and more as guidelines to be followed or disregarded as you please.

Although I have taken a few cooking classes, I am not a formally trained chef, simply a self-taught home cook who has decided that, if I'm going to eat my way to good health, it might as well be a delicious, enjoyable experience. That's why I have put together this recipe collection. I have tested these recipes on my family and friends, my children and *their* friends, and am happy to report that they've gone down well. I hope you will agree!

Chapter Three

A Cancer Epidemic

There are two facts about cancer that I never tire of repeating.

One: no one is immune to cancer. We all have cancer cells in our bodies, but only some of us develop the disease. The food we eat, our level of physical activity, the chemicals we are exposed to and our response to physical and emotional stress influences whether these cancer cells become life-threatening tumors or whether our defenses can overcome them without outside intervention.

Two: cancer is not primarily a hereditary disease. Genetic factors contribute to an estimated 5-10% of cancer cases, and even in people with a genetically heightened cancer risk, what they eat and how they lead their lives can significantly influence whether they will develop the disease or not.

So the news is both bad and good: we are all at risk of developing cancer, but it is not a preordained fate that we must bow to resignedly. The sooner we understand this, the better armed we are to fight this disease.

This chapter discusses various food-related factors that may increase our cancer risk; chapter 4 will look at ways in which the food we eat may protect us.

Boosting our defenses

Usually, a tumor starts developing in one part of the body. As it grows, it can spread to other organs or tissues, forming metastases that can disrupt their functioning. It often takes years – in some cases decades – for wide-spread cancer to develop and to show clinical symptoms. At this stage, it can be life-threatening and often requires heavy medical intervention with potentially serious side-effects.

Because cancer develops slowly through a series of stages (from "initiation" via "promotion" and "progression" to metastatic cancer) we can intervene at various points along the way to try to stop the process. So while we cannot prevent the formation of cancer cells, we can adopt lifestyle patterns, such as a healthy diet, regular physical activity, stress-reduction strategies and restful sleep, to help prevent them from becoming life-threatening.

The human body is equipped with a complex array of mechanisms designed to halt the progression of damaged cells into dangerous tumors. Our first lines of defense are the immune and lymph systems, which are equipped to identify and destroy undesirable elements like cancer cells.

Our immune system can only do its job when we are optimally nourished. Many nutrients, including vitamins A, C, E, the B-vitamins and the minerals selenium, zinc, manganese and copper, are vitally important for a well-functioning immune system. Non-nutritional factors can also boost our immunity, including regular physical activity, adequate rest and relaxation, support from family and friends and a positive outlook on life.

Inflammation, cancer's helper

The immune system works hand-in-hand with another key mechanism: inflammation. Inflammation is the body's healthy response to trauma of any kind: as soon as the immune system registers an injury, inflammation responses are triggered to repair the damage.

While this is generally a good thing, frequent or long-term inflammation increases cancer risks because it can trigger the production of cancer cells and sustain their growth and spread throughout the body. Inflammation also blocks apoptosis (a process of programmed cell death when a cell is no longer needed). Blocking apoptosis allows cancer cells to reproduce unchecked. Lastly, chronic inflammation can induce angiogenesis (the growth of new blood vessels to nourish a tumor).

Chronic inflammation, in which the same organ or body part is subjected to low-level irritation year-in, year-out increases the risk of various cancers, including cervical cancer (through infection with the human papilloma virus), stomach cancer (through infection with the bacterium Helicobacter pylori) or esophageal cancer (due to inflammation of the gullet due to repeated stomach-acid reflux).

Several factors can exacerbate inflammation, including physical and emotional stress, lack of exercise or sleep and pollutants like tobacco. However, a key factor in inflammation is diet. Deficiencies in specific nutrients such as vitamins A, folic acid, B12, C, iron, selenium and zinc may result in a failure to control inflammation. Moreover, certain types of fat, sugar and highly refined carbohydrates are thought to fuel inflammation. Other foods, including certain spices, herbs, vegetables, fruits and healthy fats, are thought to have anti-inflammatory effects.

The antioxidant defense shield

A further source of cancer risk are dangerous molecules called free oxidizing radicals, which attack and damage the membranes of our cells and the genetic information in the DNA, leading to faulty cell replication and eventually cancer.

Some free radicals arise from the body's normal metabolic functions; for instance, our immune cells purposefully create them to neutralize viruses and bacteria. Pollution, chemical toxins, radiation, cigarette smoke and pesticides in our environment also create free radicals. Food sources of free radicals include burnt, barbecued or smoked food and rancid oils.

Free radicals can be neutralized by antioxidants, which are either enzymes produced by our bodies or nutrients found in many whole foods. Antioxidant nutrients include vitamins A, C, E, the members of the carotene family, the minerals selenium, copper, zinc and manganese and a variety of other plant chemicals. All these compounds are particularly prevalent in plant foods – vegetables and fruits, nuts and seeds. They work best as a team as they support each other's functions, highlighting the need for a diet rich in a wide variety of natural foods. However, it is best to avoid environmental and food sources of free radicals as much as possible; eating antioxidants will not undo all of the damage.

Food: the double-edged sword

Almost every one of us has been touched by cancer, either because we have the disease ourselves or because a family member, a friend, a co-worker or an acquaintance has suffered or died from it.

Worldwide, 7.9 million people died of cancer in 2007, and this toll is set to rise to 13.2 million in 2030, the World Health Organization predicts[1]. Without prevention, one in two men and one in three women living in the industrialized west will eventually develop some form of cancer[2]. Cancer has become a veritable epidemic.

Epidemics don't come out of nowhere; they often accompany shifts in people's living circumstances. Western industrialized nations, in particular, have witnessed significant lifestyle changes during the last 70 years that have been accompanied by rising cancer rates. Rising cancer statistics are in part due to the increased use of sophisticated screening tests that manage to detect cancers at an early stage (when, thankfully, they are easier to treat). Increased life expectancy also contributes to rising cancer rates, for the older we are, the more prone we are to developing cancer.

However, cancer has also been increasing among young people: between 1978 and 1997, cancer incidence among European children and adolescents rose by 1.1% and 2% per year, respectively[3-4] - obviously not related to old age! And in countries like India or China, which have traditionally had significantly lower cancer rates than the industrialized west, the incidence of some types of cancer is increasing as economic development there progresses and people adopt more western lifestyles and diets.

Many aspects of western lifestyles have changed dramatically since World War Two, but one of the most significant changes over the last 70 years has been in the food we eat.

In an ideal world, food should give us energy, help us grow and maintain healthy tissues, and protect us from disease. By eating a wide variety of nourishing, natural foods brimming with essential nutrients – what scientists call a nutrient-dense diet – we feed our bodies the wide range of elements they need to maintain health.

If, however, our food provides a large number of calories derived from sugar or unhealthy fats that are not accompanied by vital nutrients (so-called empty calories), our bodies will become depleted of essential health factors. Years of nutritional impoverishment can lead to chronic diseases like cancer. Alas, 57% of the calories consumed in western societies are largely "empty", coming from refined sugar, flour and industrially processed vegetable oils[5].

Cancer cells thrive on sugar

A major shift in the western diet has been the sharp rise in refined sugar and grain intake over the last 200 years. In the US, the annual consumption of refined sugar grew from 11 pounds (5 kilos) per person in the 1830s to around 155 pounds (70 kilos) in 2000[6]. In the European Union, sugar consumption stood at 90 pounds (41.2 kilos) per person per year in 2008[7].

Eating refined carbohydrates may increase our cancer risk in several ways. For one, sugar and refined grain products contribute to weight gain, especially when coupled with the sedentary lifestyle typical of many westerners. As scientists have found, body fatness is a cause of cancers of the esophagus, pancreas, colon and rectum, breast (post-menopause), endometrium and kidney[8].

Moreover, eating sugar and refined carbohydrates triggers the production of hormones that may promote cancer. When we eat sugar or refined flour our blood-sugar (glucose) level rises. To stabilize glucose levels, our pancreas produces a hormone called insulin. Not only does insulin act as a growth factor for tumor cell proliferation, it is accompanied by the release of another hormone, called insulin-like growth factor-1 (IGF-1), that is thought to further stimulate cell growth[9] and inhibit apoptosis.

Epidemiological evidence for a link between blood glucose and cancer is mixed. Some studies have found a link between breast cancer risk and diets high in sugar and refined starch, especially in women who undertake no vigorous physical activity[10-12]. For instance, one study[13] found a 30-40% lower incidence of colon or rectal cancers in people eating a low-sugar diet, while another suggested that the risk of ovarian cancer could be cut by up to 70% by eating this type of diet[14].

Most recently, a large-scale European study suggested that having high blood sugar levels may increase the risk of several different types of cancer, independently of body weight[14a].

Other observational studies have found no association between overall dietary glycemic index or dietary glycemic load and cancer risk[15-18]. Nonetheless, since the glucose-insulin link appears - at least theoretically - to favor cancer development, because sugar and refined carbohydrates promote obesity and because they do not provide useful nutrients, it is best to limit their intake wherever possible.

Carbohydrates: the body's favorite fuel

Of course we don't need to give up carbohydrates altogether, as some weight-loss gurus recommend. They are a useful source of energy and help to fuel the proper functioning of our bodies, especially the brain. However, some types of carbohydrate are valuable health promoters while others undermine our health.

Healthy carbohydrates are found in fresh vegetables and fruits, legumes and whole, unprocessed grains. They supply energy, vitamins, minerals, water and a wide array of important plant chemicals. Vegetables, fruits, legumes and whole grains are also the body's main source of fiber, which helps balance blood-sugar levels and keeps the digestive system in healthy working order.

Less nutritious carbohydrates, such as white sugar, white flour, white pasta, white rice and concentrated fruit juices, have been transformed from their natural, whole state into a refined version that keeps longer, looks cleaner, takes less time to cook, and often tastes sweeter, but has lost most of its nutritional value.

All carbohydrates are handled the same way in the body: digestion breaks them down into blood glucose, the main energy source for the body's cells. Whole, unprocessed carbohydrates are an excellent fuel source. Because they contain protein, fats and fiber, the body only gradually converts them into glucose and this helps sustain steady energy levels for many hours. Imagine a great, dense oak log burning slowly on a fire, producing few flames but steady heat for hours – that's the equivalent of a nutrient-dense whole carbohydrate slowly releasing its energy in your body.

Refined carbohydrates, by contrast, burn much faster because they have been stripped of all nutrients except energy (calories). They resemble tissue paper that flares bright and hot for a few seconds, only to die out quickly, constantly requiring more paper to keep the fire burning. Various sugary foods and baked goods made with white flour can cause fast, sharp increases in blood sugar and, consequently, insulin. These include foods sometimes mistakenly thought of as healthy, such as energy drinks, rice crackers, bagels, corn flakes or baked potatoes.

In the 1980s, scientists devised a ranking system, the Glycemic Index (GI) that classifies carbohydrates according to the effect they have on blood glucose. Foods with a high GI value (70 or over) generally cause sharp spikes in glucose and insulin. Foods with a low GI ranking (50 or below) are absorbed more slowly, causing a less pronounced increase in glucose and insulin. A GI between 50 and 70 is moderate.

This system was further refined in the late 1990s when experts devised the concept of Glycemic Load (GL). Foods with a GL above 20 have a high glycemic impact while those below 10 are considered low-glycemic; those in-between are considered moderately glycemic.

GI and GL are a useful way of assessing whether a food is likely to cause a sharp increase in glucose, insulin and IGF-1[19]. Eating carbohydrates with low or moderate GI and GL ratings is the best way to maintain steady glucose, insulin and IGF-1 levels. (See table on pp. 42–3 for the GI and GL values of commonly eaten foods.)

The fats we eat

Many modern farm animals share a similar fate to ours: they lead sedentary lives, eat high-calorie foods not adapted to their nutritional needs and survive in crowded living conditions thanks to regular doses of antibiotics.

After World War Two, farming methods became increasingly intensive in an effort to boost yields and provide plentiful meat, eggs and dairy after years of wartime deprivation. However, in their quest for yield and efficiency, agricultural policy-makers and farmers paid less and less attention to the nutritional value of the food they were producing. As a result, many animal foods no longer provide the nutrients they previously offered, and which our bodies need.

GI and GL values of commonly eaten carbohydrate-rich foods

Food	GI	GL	Serving size (g or ml)
Bread, baked goods			
Baguette, white	95	14	30
White wheat bread	73	11	30
Whole wheat bread	68	7	30
Pizza, cheese	60	16	30
Pita, white	57	10	30
Pita, whole wheat	56	8	30
Sourdough wheat bread	54	8	30
Sourdough rye bread	48	6	30
Pasta, rice and grains			
Sushi rice	85	33	150
White rice	73	30	150
Brown rice	66	22	150
Long grain rice	56	24	150
Basmati, white	57	23	150
Couscous grains	69	23	150
Buckwheat noodles	58	25	150
Quinoa grains	53	13	150
Sweet corn, canned	46	13	150
Spaghetti, white	42	20	180
Spaghetti, whole wheat	42	17	180
Barley, hulled, boiled	22	9	150
Breakfast cereals			
Kellogg's cornflakes	93	23	30
Kellogg's Rice Krispies	82	22	30
Instant oat porridge	83	18	250
Kellogg's Special K	69	14	30
Porridge, rolled oats	42	9	250
Muesli (Alpen)	59	11	30
Oats, raw	59	11	30
Fruit: fresh, canned and dried (values vary according to degree of ripeness)			
Banana, raw	42-62	11-16	120
Dates, dried	31-62	14-21	60
Cherries, raw	63	9	120
Mango, raw	41-60	9	120
Pineapple, raw	51-66	6-8	120
Grapes, black	59	11	120
Raisins, dried	66	28	60
Apricot, raw	34-57	3-5	120
Apricot, dried	30	8	60
Apple, raw	28-44	4-6	120
Pear, raw	34-42	4-5	120
Watermelon, raw	72-80	4-5	120
Cantaloupe, raw	65-70	4	120
Orange, raw	31-51	3-6	120
Peach, raw	28-56	4-5	120
Plum, raw	25-53	3-6	120
Prunes, dried	29	10	60
Wild blueberries, raw	54	5	120
Strawberries, raw	40	1	120
Dairy products and non-dairy "milk"			
Milk, whole	34	4	250
Milk, semi-skim	34	4	250
Milk, skim	48	6	250

Food	GI	GL	Serving size (g or ml)
Soy milk, plain	44	8	250
Rice milk	79-92	17-29	250
Yogurt, plain, fat-free	35	12	200
Yogurt, strawberry, fat-free	61	18	200
Ice cream, chocolate	68	10	50
Beans and legumes (pulses)			
Red kidney beans, boiled	51	12	150
Baked beans, canned	40	6	150
Navy/haricot beans, boiled	31	9	150
Garbanzos, boiled	31	9	150
Black beans, boiled	30	7	150
Lentils, green, boiled	22	1	150
Lentils, red, boiled	18-31	3-6	150
Soy beans, boiled	15	1	150
Hummus (garbanzo dip)	6	0	30
Starchy vegetables and tubers			
Instant mashed potato	97	19	150
Potato, white, boiled	96	24	150
Potato baked (without skin)	93	17	150
Mashed potato	83	17	150
Potato boiled, refrigerated 24h, eaten cold with vinegar and olive oil	67	13	150
Beet, boiled	64	4	80
French fries	64	21	150
Potato baked with skin	69	19	150
Nicola potato w. peel, boiled	58	9	150
Carrots, raw	16	1	80
Carrots, cooked	33-49	2	80
Sweet potato, boiled	44	11	150
Pumpkin, butternut, boiled	51	3	80
Drinks			
Gatorade, orange	89	13	250
Fanta	68	23	250
Beer	66	5	250
Coca cola	63	16	250
Lemonade	54	15	250
Orange juice	46	12	250
Apple juice	44	13	250
Carrot juice	43	10	250
Snacks			
Mars bar	68	27	60
Snickers bar	68	23	60
Marshmallows	62	24	30
Potato chips	60	12	50
Twix bar	44	17	60
Plain chocolate	49	14	50
Dark chocolate	23	6	50
Tortilla chips	72	21	50
Sweeteners			
Glucose	100	10	10
Sucrose (table sugar)	60	6	10
Honey	35-87	6-18	10
Acacia honey	32	7	20
Fructose	11	1	10
Agave syrup	11	1	10

Source: University of Sydney, Australia; The Glycemic Index Foundation, www.glycemicindex.com

For example, when freely grazing cows eat grass – especially during spring – they obtain from it a class of healthy fats called omega-3 fatty acids. These fats make their way into their milk and the cheese, butter, cream or yogurt derived from it. Omega-3 fats are also found abundantly in the meat of grass-fed cattle and in eggs from free-range chickens that have eaten worms, grass and forage, rather than just grains.

Over the past 50 years, however, demand for affordable milk, meat, eggs and poultry was such that farmers had to find ways to speed up production. Pastures were replaced by more efficient battery farming. Alas, corn and soy – the staple diet of many intensively reared farm animals – contain few omega-3 fatty acids; they are rich in omega-6 fats, which, when eaten in excess, contribute to a multitude of health problems. As a result, the composition of fats in intensively reared animals has shifted. Their milk, meat and eggs may *taste* the same as that of their pastured counterparts, but the fatty acid balance in these foods has changed significantly, to our detriment.

Animal fats: the essential balance

Our bodies work best when the fats we eat contain the correct balance of two types of essential fatty acids, omega-6 and omega-3. When we eat animal products, the amount of omega-6 and omega-3 fatty acids we obtain from them depends on what the cows and chickens we eat were fed. In the succinct words of health writer Michael Pollan: "You are what you eat eats, too."[20]

Humans need to consume roughly similar amounts of omega-6 and omega-3 fats (the relationship between the two is called the omega-6-to-3 ratio)[21]. This is reflected in the composition of human milk with its omega-6-to-3 ratio of around 2:1 (two times more omega-6 fats than omega-3), considered the ideal ratio to sustain human health[22].

However, most people eating a western diet consume significantly more omega-6 fats than omega-3, and this can be a problem. Among others, omega-6 fatty acids have an inflammation-fueling effect that encourages cancer cells to grow and spread. Omega-3 fats, on the other hand, can reduce inflammation. They are also thought to enhance the effects of certain types of chemotherapy and radiation treatments, slow tumor growth, and reduce the risk of wasting (cachexia) in cancer patients.

The omega-6-to-3 ratios of meat, dairy and eggs from animals raised on modern feed are far away from the ideal 2:1 balance. While eggs from free-roaming hens eating insects and green plants contain an omega-6-to-3 ratio of approximately 2:1, mass-produced commercial eggs can contain as much as 20 times more omega-6 than omega-3 (20:1)![23]

Meanwhile, a recent investigation comparing the milks of intensively reared and pastured cows in Denmark showed that pasture-fed cows produced milk with a high concentration antioxidant vitamins (beta carotene and vitamin E) and an omega-6-to-omega-3 ratio of 1 (i.e. equal amounts of omega-6 and omega-3). By contrast, conventionally reared cows fed a commercial mix of rapeseed, soybean meal and maize silage produced milk with between 30% and 60% fewer antioxidant vitamins and an omega-6-to-3 ratio of 4.7 (nearly five times more omega-6 fats than omega-3) [24].

The shift to modern feeding methods hasn't only upset the natural omega-6-to-3 balance in our diets; it has also led to a decline in the conjugated linoleic acid (CLA) available from dairy products. CLA, a type of fat found mainly in the milk, cheese and butter of grass-fed cows and in eggs, is thought to lower cancer risk. Animal and laboratory investigations indicate that it may reduce the risk of numerous types of cancers, including breast, prostate, colorectal, stomach[25] and brain[26].

In a recent British study, milk from pasture-fed cows was shown to contain up to twice as much CLA as that of conventionally fed cows, 39% more omega-3 fatty acids, 50% more vitamin E and 80% more carotenoids, both of which are antioxidant nutrients[27].

Unhealthy processed vegetable fats

The animal fats in our diet are not the only ones that have undergone dramatic changes. Since World War Two there has also been a sharp rise in the consumption of margarine and partially hydrogenated vegetable fats.

To become hydrogenated, seed oils undergo a chemical reaction at high temperature that makes them solid. Partially hydrogenated fats are usually made from oils rich in inflammatory omega-6 fats such as sunflower, safflower, corn or soy oil.

In addition to their high levels of omega-6 fats, partially hydrogenated fats also contain a type of fatty acid called trans fat that results from hydrogenation. Trans fats are thought to further increase inflammation and block the body's ability to use healthy fats such as omega-3 fatty acids.

Man-made margarines and vegetable shortenings are widely used in industrial food processing (ready meals, bread and baked goods, snack foods, etc.). The benefit to industrial food producers of using these fats is that they are cheap to make and more stable than unprocessed plant oils; thus, they can better resist the deleterious effects of heat and light that cause natural oils to go rancid. They also give processed foods a longer shelf life and a less greasy feel.

But often, the more convenient a food, the unhealthier it is. Tragically, in the 1970s and 80s many people switched from butter to margarine in the mistaken belief that this would protect them from disease. Now it appears that processed seed oils, and in particular the trans fats they contain, may have in fact helped fuel the degenerative diseases – such as heart disease and cancer – that are taking the west by storm.

A toxic environment

In addition to our deteriorating food quality, we are increasingly exposed to man-made chemicals. The production of synthetic chemicals has increased sharply in the last 70 years, from 1 million tons in 1930 to 400 million tons in 2001[28]. About 100,000 different synthetic chemicals are currently in use, but for most of these the potential risks to human health are unknown.

Many of these chemicals are in the food we eat, via pesticide or herbicide residues, in kitchen ware and food packaging materials and in artificial additives. They are in the air we breathe, the clothes we wear, the soft furnishings in our homes and offices, the cosmetics we put on our skin and the water we drink.

Some say that worries about the health risks of man-made chemicals are exaggerated and unnecessarily alarmist. They argue that tobacco smoking, infections and obesity caused by poor food choices and sedentary lifestyles carry much greater cancer risks than agricultural or domestic chemicals.

Certainly, smoking, infections and obesity are important risk factors, but synthetic chemicals may play a role as well. It took several decades for the link between smoking and cancer to become accepted; toxic pesticides such as DDT and Lindane were once considered safe by regulators, only to be banned when their health risks became apparent. Maybe 20 years from now, we will better understand the possible contribution of man-made chemicals to rising cancer rates.

Pesticide residues in food

The use of synthetic pesticides and herbicides in agriculture has increased sharply in the last 60 years. Nearly 2,500 tons of these chemicals were used worldwide in 2001[29].

Direct exposure, through touch or inhalation, to pesticides around the home and in agriculture increases the risk of cancer. People who are in close contact with pesticides should use protective clothing and masks, and the use of synthetic pesticides in homes and gardens should be avoided.

Pesticide exposure through food is a less clear-cut issue and a subject of controversy. In 2007, of the 11,683 samples of fresh and processed foods tested by the US Department of Agriculture, 77% contained traces of at least one pesticide and 46 different residues were detected in treated drinking water[30].

Defenders of farming methods that allow the use of synthetic pesticides argue that, where residues are present, it is in infinitesimally small doses deemed safe by regulators. They also note that the human body is equipped with detoxification capacities that allow it to eliminate natural and man-made toxins.

However, critics of agrichemicals warn that in the presence of ever-increasing amounts of environmental toxins, even modest pesticide residues may pose risks, especially to fetuses and children. While the amounts of residual chemicals on produce may be small, they warn that growers often use several different products on the same crops and it is not known how this cocktail of chemicals may affect our health.

According to the WCRF/AICR, there is no epidemiological evidence that current pesticide exposures cause cancer in humans. However, its Expert Report recommends a "precautionary approach … for women of reproductive age, since vulnerability during embryonic phases of development is increased and early exposure may result in increased risk at later stages in life."

Some people prefer to err on the safe side by switching to organically produced food, which is less likely to contain pesticide residues than produce grown with the use of agrichemicals.

To be sure, people eating organic food ingest fewer pesticides than those who eat non-organically grown produce. In a study of children fed either organic or conventionally grown food for three days, researchers measuring the level of organochlorine pesticides in the children's urine found that the level of pesticides in the urine of the "organic" children was well below the maximum set by the US Environmental Protection Agency, and was one-sixth of that of the "non-organic" children. Meanwhile, in some of the children eating non-organic foods, the level of pesticides was four times over the official safety limit[31].

Some fruits and vegetables are more likely to contain pesticide residues than others. For instance, those with large, leafy surfaces that chemical spray residues can cling to (such as cabbage, spinach or lettuce), or those whose skin we consume (such as apples or grapes), may be more significant dietary sources of pesticides.

Since fruits and vegetables account for the majority of pesticide residues in the diet, especially the diets of babies and children, it is important to know which are the most affected.

The US Environmental Working Group (EWG) on its website publishes data on pesticide residues found on 50 popular fruits and vegetables based on an analysis of 89,000 tests for pesticides on these foods, conducted from 2000 to 2008 by the U.S. Department of Agriculture and the federal Food and Drug Administration (www.foodnews.org/fulllist.php)[32].

According to the EWG, the 10 *most contaminated vegetables* tested were celery (worst), sweet bell peppers, spinach, kale or collard greens, potatoes, lettuce, carrots, domestic green beans, summer squash and imported cucumbers. The *least contaminated vegetables* were onions (best), frozen sweet corn, sweet peas, asparagus, cabbage, eggplant, sweet potatoes, winter squash, broccoli and tomatoes.

Among fruits, the *highest levels* of pesticide residues were found in peaches, strawberries, apples, domestic blueberries, nectarines, cherries, imported grapes, imported blueberries and pears. The *least contaminated fruits* were pineapples, mango, kiwi fruit, cantaloupe, watermelon, grapefruit, honeydew melon, domestic plums, cranberries and bananas.

In publicizing these findings I do not in any way wish to discourage you from eating fresh fruits and vegetables – they are among the best sources of natural anti-cancer compounds available, and the benefits of regularly eating a wide variety of plant foods outweigh the possible side effects of any pesticide residues.

However, if you are concerned about pesticide residues, you can use the EWG findings to help you minimize potential exposure. For instance, you could replace produce in the "most contaminated" list with organic equivalents while increasing your consumption of fruit and vegetables in the "least contaminated" list. You could also make your concerns about pesticide residues known to your local supermarket. Lastly, if you have a garden, why not grow pesticide-free fruits and vegetables yourself?

The meat we eat

The best way to optimize our diets is to be informed, discerning consumers: understanding dietary risk factors can help us make healthier choices. An area where many of these risk factors come together is meat.

For years, scientists have been debating the role of meat in cancer development. The World Cancer Research Fund/American Institute for Cancer Research (WCRF/ AICR) in its 2007 Expert Report[33] concluded that "red meat is a convincing cause of colorectal cancer," adding that it might also be a cause of esophageal, pancreatic and endometrial cancer.

The WCRF/AICR also found processed meat (i.e., meat preserved by salting, curing, smoking or the addition of preservatives such as nitrites) to be a "convincing cause" of colorectal cancer and said there was limited evidence that it contributes to esophageal, lung, stomach and prostate cancer.

What exactly causes the risks of meat-eating remains unclear; indeed, it may be a complex interaction of factors.

The presence of iron in red meat may be one risk factor. Although the body needs iron to maintain healthy blood cells, excessive levels may cause free-radical damage. Red meat and organ meats such as liver, liver paté and blood sausage are the main sources of iron in the human diet; by contrast, chicken and fish contain little iron.

One way of reducing the risks posed by iron is to accompany a red-meat meal with foods high in calcium as this mineral lowers the absorption of iron from food – for instance, eating a small piece of cheese or a yogurt after eating red meat. Certain compounds in red wine or green tea are also known to bind to iron and may limit its potential to cause harm.

Meanwhile, preserved meats such as cold cuts, sausage or bacon often contain added nitrites. Sodium or potassium nitrite is used for the curing of meat because it prevents bacterial growth and gives the product an appetizing red color. Under certain conditions, nitrites in meat are transformed into so-called nitrosamines that may contribute to the development of certain cancers, especially in the stomach.

Antioxidants, particularly vitamins C and E, and sulfur compounds found in garlic can inhibit the conversion of sodium nitrite into nitrosamines; they are particularly prevalent in plant food such as fruits, vegetables, nuts and seeds, which may be the reason why a diet rich in fruits and vegetables has been shown to protect humans against several forms of cancer. The fiber in vegetables and fruit also speeds up intestinal transit, giving potentially harmful substances from meat less contact time with the mucous membranes lining the gut, another way of reducing cancer risk.

Cooking methods are a further potential source of health risks arising from meat. When meat is barbecued, fried or grilled at high temperatures, potentially carcinogenic substances are produced. During barbecuing, fat drippings create smoke containing carcinogenic polycyclic aromatic hydrocarbons (PAHs). As the smoke envelops the food, it transfers the PAHs onto the surface of the meat. Using wood to barbecue meat causes more heat, and thus more PAHs, than using charcoal.

When red meat, chicken and fish are fried or barbecued at high temperatures, compounds inside the food may create another harmful substance, heterocyclic amines (HCAs). HCAs, which may increase the risk of colorectal, stomach, lung, pancreatic, breast and prostate cancers in humans, are found in muscle meats such as beef, pork, fowl, and fish cooked above 300°F (150°C).

Other sources of protein (milk, eggs, tofu, and organ meats such as liver) produce no HCAs when cooked. Oven roasting and baking involve lower temperatures so fewer HCAs are likely to form, though gravy made from meat drippings contains substantial amounts. Stewing, boiling or poaching takes place at around 210°F (100°C), creating negligible amounts of HCAs.

Marinating meat with spices and herbs reduces the formation of HCAs even at high temperatures. One study showed that in beef steaks bathed for an hour in a "Caribbean" marinade containing thyme, rosemary, red and black pepper, allspice and chives and cooked at 400°F (204°C), HCA content was 88% lower than in non-marinated meat[34]. So, if you occasionally barbecue or fry meat, marinating it first may reduce the health risk of high-temperature cooking.

Smoking as a food conservation technique poses further risks. This process of exposing meat or fish to wood smoke can again generate the formation of PAHs. Lastly, salting and curing of meat and fish is also associated with increased cancer risk, notably stomach cancer[35].

Thus it seems that it is not so much "meat" *per se*, but the way it is preserved, prepared and eaten that may represent health risks. Small portions of high-quality meat - including red meat - cooked at low temperatures with the addition of herbs and spices and eaten three or four times a week along with generous portions of antioxidant-rich vegetables and fruits are less likely to be a problem than large slabs of barbecued or processed meat from intensively eared animals eaten with French fries and factory-made mayonnaise!

Speaking of French fries and high-temperature food preparation techniques, there is one more risk factor not related to meat: acrylamide. This substance is found in processed foods such as potato chips and extruded salty snacks, processed breakfast cereals, French fries, bread, crisp breads and also soluble coffee or substitute coffee drinks.

Although there is mixed evidence as to the possible link between acrylamide and human cancer, the compound has been found to cause cancer in laboratory animals and so efforts should be made to minimize exposure from all sources including diet, according to the European Food Safety Authority.

Another diet-related risk factor emanates from so-called aflatoxins, toxic substances produced by certain moulds or fungi that can cause liver cancer. Aflatoxins can be found on cereal grains, legumes, seeds and nuts (especially peanuts) stored in warm, damp conditions. According to the WCRF/AICR, exposure levels are low in Europe and Australia, higher in the US and high in many low-income countries – especially tropical regions with a warm, damp climate, poor storage facilities and incomplete aflatoxin monitoring.

To reduce potential aflatoxin exposure, buy grains and nuts (particularly corn or peanuts) from reputable sources, store them in a dry, cool place (ideally the refrigerator or freezer) and do not keep them for more than a few months before eating.

Beware of plastic linings

One chemical that has been getting a lot of bad press is bisphenol-A (BPA). It is used to make plastic containers and the linings that coat the insides of food and drink cans.

BPA is thought to act as a "xenoestrogen" – a substance that acts like estrogen and thereby may stimulate hormone receptors on cell membranes, especially in the estrogen-sensitive tissues of prostate and breast. Moreover, even at weak concentrations BPA has been shown to block the effects of several commonly used chemotherapy agents on breast cancer cells[36].

But BPA isn't the only xenoestrogen in our food: the vast majority of plastics currently used in food processing – whether it's in the linings of food or soft-drink cans, plastic food wrap and sandwich bags, disposable water bottles, children's sippy cups, airtight food storage containers, convenience-food packaging or kitchen appliances (espresso makers, kettles, water filters, etc.) – contain chemical compounds that leach into the foods we eat, and which can have adverse health effects. Indeed, some of these are through to have even stronger xeno-estrogenic properties than BPA!

In a recent US-government funded investigation[37], a research team from Texas found that 92% of all BPA-free kitchen plastics tested leached these compounds into food they came into contact with, even when they were not being stressed (e.g. exposed to heat or light). Under stress, some 98% of plastics gave off these compounds.

Experts disagree at which concentrations BPA may be dangerous; until more is known about safe levels of BPA, the precautionary principle should prevail and humans - especially women of childbearing age and young children - are best off minimizing their exposure to BPA. Here are some ways to do this:

• Instead of buying food that's tightly packaged in plastic (e.g. cheese or cold cuts from a supermarket chiller cabinet), buy it loose (e.g. at a deli counter, loosely wrapped in paper) and store in glass or stainless steel containers at home. Use these also for leftovers or fresh foods stored in fridge and freezer.

- Instead of buying food in tins, eat fresh food, or can it yourself in glass jars. (Some food manufacturers use BPA-free tins; these can make useful pantry staples.) The lids of many glass jars are also lined with plastic, so choose a brand that doesn't have these (e.g. Weck, which uses glass lids and a natural latex rubber seal). They also make attractive storage containers for dry foods (e.g. beans, nuts, rice) in cupboards and on shelves (their tight seals keep out food mites!).
- Babies should drink from glass bottles; toddlers can use stainless steel sippy cups. Their food should be heated in non-reactive materials such as glass or porcelain (if using a microwave oven) or stainless steel. Canned formula or foods should be avoided.
- Drink filtered water from stainless-steel bottles instead of plastic ones (especially if these have been exposed to sunlight). Avoid drinks in cans, which are lined with plastic resins.
- Use ceramic, glass or metal bowls to prepare food. This is especially important if you use a microwave oven. For cooking, use stainless steel or cast iron pots and pans and wooden, bamboo or stainless steel implements (spoons, spatulas, strainers, etc.) instead of plastics.
- At the dining table, use china or earthenware plates, and pitchers and glasses made of glass, not plastic.
- Instead of a plastic water kettle, use an old-fashioned enamel or stainless steel stove-top kettle.
- Instead of automatic espresso machines, opt for a stainless steel stovetop espresso maker. If you make drip-filtered coffee, use paper filters in a ceramic, glass or stainless steel filter holder, rather than plastic equivalents.

And now for the good news!

After reading this chapter, you'll be forgiven for feeling despondent. But despair not! There are many simple ways to avoid the risks described here and still enjoy eating and drinking.

Granted, when you start to replace old dietary habits with new ones you may feel confused by so much change. However, most people quickly come to grips with the dietary and lifestyle changes recommended here, so much so that before long, the changes become new, self-reinforcing habits.

Chapter 4 aims to help you make this transition as smoothly as possible. It describes ways to replace unhealthy sugars and fats with healthy ones, how to increase your intake of healthy vegetables and fruits and how to diminish your exposure to potentially hazardous substances. You'll see – it's all quite feasible. Just take it one step at a time.

Chapter Four

Eating For Life

Some 2,500 years ago in ancient Greece, Hippocrates, the founding father of modern medicine, coined the dictum: "Let food be thy medicine." He, too, may have been inspired by the health benefits of the Mediterranean diet he was eating daily!

Having described in the previous chapter how some foods can make us sick, let's take a look at the many delicious ways food can keep us healthy.

Let's be clear: there is no single miracle food that can "cure cancer," nor can healthy foods alone prevent the disease; healthy body weight, regular exercise, not smoking, restful sleep, psychological well-being and other factors are important too. Yet a diet based on a wide variety of fresh, natural foods – mostly from plant sources – provides a range of nutrients that help protect us from cancer.

Bolstering our defenses

Due to normal physiological processes, most of us produce and carry microscopically small tumors in our bodies about which we are unaware. In many cases, our bodies' defense systems nip these micro-tumors in the bud and stop them from growing, but when our defenses are disturbed, they can develop into life-threatening cancers. This is where food may help.

Some call this "nutritional chemoprevention," a process in which a wide range of anti-cancer agents of nutritional – rather than pharmaceutical – origin, ingested repeatedly throughout the day, every day, may protect us from cancer by shielding our cells from free-radical damage and removing toxins from the body. Even when micro-tumors are already present, certain compounds in our food may prompt cancer cells to self-destruct or may prevent their progression into malignant tumors.

Thus, by eating a natural, nutrient-rich diet we may create an environment that is hostile to the development of invasive tumors. Some liken this to an "on-off" switch[1]: in people eating a diet lacking cancer-protective nutrients, this diet acts as an "on" switch for cancer and creates a terrain that encourages their growth and spread. On the other hand, in people eating a diet rich in protective foods and low in cancer-fueling foods, micro-tumors cannot thrive and the risk of developing full-blown cancer is reduced: the switch is turned "off."

Cancer is a complex condition that undergoes various stages of development, often over a long period. No single food possesses all the molecules needed to act on all the stages of development. Some foods, such as cabbage or citrus fruit, assist the body in eliminating toxic molecules that could trigger the development of cancerous cells. Others, such as green tea, berries or soy, may act at a later stage by preventing the formation of new blood vessels needed for tumors to grow. A few – such as red and blue berries – are thought to intervene at nearly every stage of cancer development.

This chapter does not offer a list of "proven anti-cancer foods." Given the uncertainty that prevails in many areas of nutritional science, no book could responsibly do so. In-depth research into many of the foods featured here suggests that they may boost our defenses against cancer, but definitive proof eludes scientists, for various reasons.

Much of the research into dietary cancer prevention is carried out on cell cultures in test tubes or on small laboratory animals. While such studies may yield positive results, it is not certain that these can be replicated in humans: the same compound eaten by fully grown people living in the real world may not have the same effect as it does on laboratory mice or cells in test tubes.

So why don't we study foods and their effects on real-live people? Human intervention studies measuring the effects of certain foods on human health are tricky. For one, they are long, labor intensive and very expensive.

Moreover, because humans are complex beings with highly varied food and lifestyle habits, the results of intervention studies may be hard to interpret. For it is difficult to control humans' food intake and lifestyle factors for the prolonged period of time needed to measure the effect of, say, a person's cocoa consumption on their cancer risk.

Lastly, it is ethically unsound to test foods on humans that may have negative effects on their health. Moreover, if you split subjects into two groups, with one receiving a particular nutritional intervention and the other not, the group deriving the greater benefit would be at a distinct advantage over the other – another thorny ethical issue, especially when the subjects are suffering from a serious disease.

Sadly, there is little commercial incentive for studying the effects of foods and nutrients on cancer. Drug companies spend fortunes on developing medicines that can be patented and sold at a handsome profit. However, food belongs to Mother Nature and cannot be patented, thus no one studying its health effects would receive a return on their investment.

Pointless until proven effective?

Because the cancer-preventive or therapeutic properties of many foods are not proven beyond doubt, some skeptics say that people should not be encouraged to eat certain foods in the hope of preventing or overcoming cancer.

To be sure, I do not advocate food as a cancer treatment once the disease has declared itself and I urge cancer patients to follow their doctors' treatment plans. I also do not advocate one-sided regimes resting heavily on a handful of so-called "anti-cancer foods" to the exclusion of other healthy foods.

Think back to the Mediterranean diet principle of "variety." Having reviewed the scientific literature, I have concluded that there is no single "miracle food;" it is the combination of many natural, fresh foods, carefully prepared and savored with pleasure, that I believe offers the best protection.

True to the maxim "if a little is good, more must be better," some people eat large volumes of foods widely thought to be cancer-protective. This is understandable; most people who are worried about a potentially life-threatening disease will do what they can to boost their defenses.

However, not only do restrictive or repetitive eating patterns crowd out other nutritious foods, they may even put your health at risk. Thus, eating large amounts of raw cabbage[2] or soy foods[3] may provoke thyroid problems. Similarly, completely avoiding animal products – such as meat, fish, eggs – can lead to protein, vitamin and essential fatty acid deficiencies[4] unless great care and nutritional supplements are taken.

Meanwhile, it is widely claimed that curcumin, the yellow pigment obtained from turmeric, is efficient and safe in the prevention and treatment of cancer. However, the evidence is far from unequivocal[5]. Thus, curcumin has been shown to both increase and reduce the efficiency of chemotherapy, depending on the concentration at which it is used[6,7]. Moreover, at high concentrations it may cause potentially carcinogenic damage to the genetic material in cells (DNA)[8] and may also block iron absorption from the diet, raising the risk of iron deficiency in people with low iron stores[9].

This is not to say that raw cabbage, soy, vegan eating patterns or turmeric should not be a part of our diets. Of course they can be – but not every day, at every meal, in large quantities. I recommend a return to nutritional common sense, meaning that we should eat *moderate amounts and a wide variety* of naturally grown, seasonal vegetables, fruits, nuts, fish and lean meat, healthy fats, herbs, spices and other delicious foods featured in this book, whilst avoiding processed, nutrient-depleted calories.

Plant power

Plant foods are among our greatest allies in the preservation of health and vitality.

Being generally high in nutrients and fiber and low in calories, they help prevent obesity. People obtaining more than 55% of their carbohydrate intake from vegetables, fruits and whole grains consume 200 to 300 fewer calories than those eating the standard western diet of refined grains, processed oils, sugar and salt, and have the lowest BMI (body mass index) scores[10]. The World Cancer Research Fund/ American Institute for Cancer Research recommends that adults keep their weight in the BMI range of 21-23.

Healthy weight has important implications for cancer prevention: for cancers of the esophagus, pancreas, gall bladder, bowel, breast, endometrium and kidney, in the US 20% of these cancers in men and 19% in women could be prevented if people had a healthy body weight, the WCRF/AICR estimates[11].

A diet rich in plant foods provides not only essential vitamins, minerals and fiber at low caloric cost, but also thousands of phytochemicals (plant chemicals) with wide-ranging health effects. These chemicals - many of which plants produce to protect themselves against predators - also have a multitude of cancer-protective properties.

As we saw in Chapter 3, free-radical attacks can damage our cells' genetic information and trigger uncontrolled cell growth. This damage can be limited by antioxidant compounds in fruits and vegetables that help detoxify the body, neutralize free radicals, stimulate the immune system and slow or even reverse cell growth. Indeed, many plant extracts may have more than one protective mechanism.

Beautiful Brassicas

Members of the cabbage family ("cruciferous vegetables," or "Brassicas") are an excellent source of plant chemicals. There is a vast array of Brassicas to choose from, from the more traditional cabbages such as white, green/Savoy and red, cauliflower, broccoli and Brussels sprouts, to less commonly eaten brassicas that include garden cress and watercress, broccoli sprouts, bok choy, daikon (Japanese radish), collard greens, mustard greens, mustard seeds, rutabaga, kohlrabi, turnips and their greens, kale, horseradish, wasabi (Japanese horseradish), radish, collards, and the spicy, leafy greens, mizuna and arugula.

Sulforaphane, the molecule that gives Brassicas their sharp taste, is thought to help eliminate toxic compounds linked to the development of cancer and may trigger the self destruction of some types of cancer cells. Among Brassicas, broccoli is the best source of sulforaphane. Sprouted broccoli seeds, sold in health-food shops but also easy to grow at home, are an even more concentrated source of this compound: they contain between 10 and 100 times more sulforaphane than fully grown broccoli[12].

Brassicas can be eaten all year round: stewed or steamed in the colder seasons and blanched or raw in the warmer months (raw cabbage has the extra advantage of soothing inflamed digestive tracts, especially when juiced). Broccoli or cauliflower can be served raw or lightly steamed with dips or in salads, or added to soups and stir fries.

Caution: Raw Brassicas may suppress thyroid function, so people with low thyroid function should avoid eating them raw. Likewise, for people who struggle to digest raw cabbage, steaming it for 2-3 minutes may make it easier to digest. To preserve their cancer-protective nutrients, Brassicas should be briefly steamed rather than boiled and cooked al dente rather than soft.

Some studies have cast doubt on vegetables' and fruits' cancer-protective qualities. For instance, one widely-reported European investigation concluded that every two portions of vegetables and fruit consumed per day conferred only a 2.5% reduction of cancer risk[13].

A casual reader of news reports about this study might have concluded that vegetables and fruits offer next-to-no protection against cancer. However, what got less attention was the finding that those study participants who were eating the most fruits and vegetables – six or more servings per day – had a nearly 11% lower risk of all cancers than those who ate the least. Thus, it may be that five portions of fruits and vegetables are simply not enough, and that more may be needed to protect us from cancer.

The study also did not assess the *variety* of fruit and vegetables eaten, only the total mass. On this basis, the participants' total fruit and vegetable intake could technically have been based on only one kind of fruit or vegetable, rather than a variety of different types. The types of vegetable and fruit eaten were also not analyzed; thus iceberg lettuce or bananas would have ranked equally with broccoli and raspberries, although the first two foods provide only a fraction of the cancer-protective nutrients of the latter two.

What may also have skewed results was that the study did not differentiate between different types of cancer, yielding a fairly flat result. When types of cancer are assessed separately, vegetables and fruits appear to have a more noticeable effect, as the table below illustrates.

Prospective studies into the link between the intake of specific foods and cancer incidence in human populations[14]

Food	Number of study participants	Type of cancer	Risk reduction
Brassicas	47 909	Bladder	50%
Brassicas	4 309	Lung	30%
Brassicas	29 361	Prostate	50%
Tomatoes	47 365	Prostate	25%
Citrus fruit	521 457	Stomach, oesophagus	25%
Green vegetables	81 922	Pancreas	75%
Green vegetables	11 699	Breast (post-menopause)	44%
Lignans	58 049	Breast (post-menopause ER+)	28%
Carrots	490 802	Head and throat	46%
Apples, pears, plums	490 802	Head and throat	38%

I therefore believe vegetables and fruits – high in nutrients, phytochemicals and fiber, low in calories – do offer significant protection and should make up a large proportion of our diet. That's why it is worrying that many people in industrialized countries don't eat nearly enough of them.

In the US, only a fifth of the population eats five portions of fruit and vegetables each day; average intake is just over three portions a day (on average, men eat 2.9

portions and women eat 3.5 portions daily)[15]. The situation is even more dismal in the UK, where only 12% of the population manages to eat five fruits or vegetables a day and nearly 40% eat one portion or less. On average, Brits eat an average of 2.5 portions of fruits and vegetables daily[16].

Greens are slightly more popular in continental Europe; French women, for example, eat on average 3.8 portions of fruits and vegetables per day, closely followed by French men at 3.4 portions a day[17]; nonetheless, even French intakes aren't enough to satisfy official five-a-day guidelines.

Amid increasing evidence that vegetables and fruits offer significant protection, health authorities in many western countries are continually increasing their recommendations for vegetable and fruit intake. The US government, for example, recently raised its recommendation to 5-13 portions a day. For people whose vegetable and fruit intake is low, bridging the gap from current low intakes to these recommended amounts will require an effort; hopefully the recipes in this book can help.

Allium allies

One of the flavors most people associate with Mediterranean cuisine comes from the allium family: garlic, onions, leeks, shallots, spring onions and chives. Organosulfur compounds such as diallyl sulphide and a flavonoid, quercetin, in alliums may help prevent the onset or progression of certain types of cancers, especially stomach, colorectal, laryngeal and esophageal cancers[18]. Garlic has anti-inflammatory, antiviral, anti-bacterial and anti-fungal effects[19], may induce cancer cells' self-destruction and prevent the formation of new blood vessels by tumors[20].

The health effects of garlic are at their most powerful when raw garlic is chopped, triggering an enzyme reaction that creates allicin, the compound that not only confers some of garlic's many health benefits, but also its pungent taste. Garlic is best chopped and left to sit for 5-10 minutes before use to optimize allicin levels.

The same applies to leeks and onions; indeed, the more finely you cut an onion and the more tear-provoking its smell, the more of these healthy compounds you will obtain. Cooking causes allicin concentrations to decline, so try to eat at least some garlic and onions raw or barely cooked.

Vegetable vigor

"Vegetables" and "fruits" usually get lumped together as mutually inter-changeable and similarly nutritious foods. It is true that both categories provide substantial health benefits. However, compared on a nutritional basis, vegetables contain a wider variety of nutrients, fewer calories and less sugar than fruits.

Modern fruit – especially the kind we buy at supermarkets – is often bred to be sweet and good-looking rather than nutritious. Research shows that wild fruits often contain more protein, higher levels of nutrients such as calcium, potassium, iron and phosphorus and healthier sugars than the cultivated varieties sold by mass retailers[21]. However, they tend to be less sweet, smaller and less visually appealing than modern cultivars.

Even modern fruits provide health benefits, however. Indeed, some fruits (such as berries) are more nutritious than some vegetables (for example, iceberg lettuce), and *any* fresh fruit is better than a candy bar!

Generally, we should aim to eat the *right kinds* of fruit (high in nutrients and with a moderate glycemic index rating), and to balance vegetables and fruits, eating slightly more of the latter than the former. For a person eating nine daily portions, five to six would ideally be vegetables and three to four fruit.

Alas, vegetables seem to be less popular than fruit. That's because fruit is more convenient to transport and easier to prepare, but particularly because its sugar content appeals to humans' innate sweet tooth. Moreover, many of us dislike vegetables as a result of being forced to eat tasteless, overcooked greens in our youth. In my cooking classes, participants' most common request is to "learn to like vegetables" and to prepare these in an appetizing, varied and fun way.

Vegetables should feature on our plates every day, at every meal. The more colorful and more strongly flavored they are, the more likely they are to provide health benefits, as the plant chemicals that give them their color and flavor are often those that boost our cancer defenses.

Five to six portions of vegetables may sound like more than most of us are used to, but it's quite easy to enjoy these throughout the day. For example, we can eat them in a Frittata (pp. 154-55) or omelet (pp. 160-162) for breakfast (using leftover vegetables to save time); in a large, mixed salad for lunch (pp. 124-135); in a vegetable soup for dinner (pp. 136-152) and raw as a snack in between meals.

Fish or meat eaten at lunch or dinner can be accompanied with vegetables rather than the much less nutritious pasta, rice or potatoes that take nearly as long to prepare. Many vegetables – such as spaghetti squash, green beans, cauliflower or spinach – are tasty substitutes for pasta and taste great with any sauce you might serve on pasta, such as Bolognese, pesto or tomato sauce.

If you learn to select and cook vegetables in the simple and tasty ways shown in this book, your taste buds will transform themselves into vegetable lovers. Give it time; it can take weeks for people who have had little exposure to good vegetables to learn to like them.

Marvelous mushrooms

Did you know that Japanese mushroom growers are nearly 50% less likely to develop stomach cancer than their non-mushroom-farming neighbors?[22] This may be due to the fact that they regularly eat the mushrooms they cultivate and benefit from the cancer-protective compounds in them.

Many mushrooms are thought to have antioxidant, anti-inflammatory, immune-system enhancing, anti-viral and possibly even direct anti-tumor effects. Shiitake mushrooms, for instance, are a rich source of lentinan, a molecule thought to stimulate the immune system and to slow or even stop tumor growth. Clinical studies of cancer patients associate lentinan with a higher survival rate, higher quality of life and lower recurrence of cancer[23-25].

The best-known medicinal mushrooms are Asian varieties such as oyster mushrooms, maitake, shiitake or reishi. Even everyday button mushrooms may have a protective effect: Researchers at Perth University found that Chinese women eating on average 4 grams of dried button mushrooms daily cut their breast cancer risk by 47% compared to women eating none, while those eating 10 grams of fresh mushrooms daily lowered their risk by 64%. Those who combined mushrooms with regular green tea intake even saw their breast-cancer risk decline by 89% [26].

Button mushrooms are thought to contain natural aromatase inhibitors, substances that can block production of estrogen in the body. This may protect against breast cancer and other cancers dependent on estrogen to grow. However, eaten raw, they also contain compounds called hydrazines, which may be carcinogenic. Hydrazines are destroyed by cooking, drying or canning, so it is best to eat mushrooms cooked, and to alternate button mushrooms and other varieties, such as oyster or shiitake mushrooms, which are increasingly available in supermarkets and health-food stores.

Which fruits are best?

Fruits are an excellent source of vitamins, minerals, water and fiber, in addition to brimming with health-promoting plant chemicals and delicious flavors. The natural sugars in fruit provide energy and are healthier than sugars derived from soft drinks, mass-manufactured cookies, crackers or candy bars.

One type of compound found mostly in fruit, pectin (a soluble fiber used as a gelling agent in jam-making), may have anti-cancer properties, notably in preventing or slowing the spread of cancer cells[27,28]. Apples, quinces, plums, gooseberries, bananas, oranges and other citrus fruits (especially citrus skin) are excellent sources of pectin, as are carrots – one of the few vegetable sources.

Berry bonanza

For a plant food that offers heady aromas, healthy plant chemicals and few calories, choose berries and stone fruits. Ellagic acid, a compound found in raspberries, strawberries and some nuts, such as hazelnuts and pecans, is thought to slow the growth and spread of tumors and aid the body in detoxifying potentially cancer-causing substances. Cherries, plums, peaches and nectarines share berries' vivid colors and high antioxidant levels; often they are also less expensive.

The best way to eat berries is fresh and raw, but since growing seasons in many parts of the world are short, frozen berries are fine too. As different types of berries contain varying types of protective compounds, the best thing is to vary the types of berries you eat, for example, selecting raspberries one day, strawberries the next and blueberries or cranberries another, and alternating between fresh, frozen and dried berries.

If you have a small garden, why not plant a few strawberry plants of your own? Strawberry and raspberry plants carry fruit year after year and require little more than some light weeding and watering, with occasional feeding of organic fertilizer or home-made compost.

The best way to eat fruit is raw, fresh and whole – the way it comes off the tree or bush. Wherever possible, choose locally grown, seasonal fruit that has ripened on the tree; it is generally fresher, tastier and less expensive than imported out-of-season fruit.

While dried fruit is an excellent source of fiber, it loses many of its vitamins during dehydration. Moreover, drying fruit concentrates its sugars and increases its calorie content. Therefore, it's best to eat mostly fresh fruit, enjoying dried fruit occasionally as a treat.

Fruit juices can cause unhealthier blood-glucose and insulin spikes than whole fruit because the fruits' fiber – from pulp, pips and skin – has been removed, allowing the sugars to convert more rapidly into blood glucose. Still, fruit juice is preferable to sugar-laden fizzy drinks and if you are trying to wean yourself off such beverages, juice can help.

When drinking juice, avoid shop-bought brands (many of which contain added sweeteners and are made from juice concentrates rather than 100% whole fruit). Instead, choose freshly pressed juice – either home-made or freshly pressed at a juice bar – and drink it immediately after pressing as the vitamins degrade quickly upon exposure to oxygen. Diluting juice with water will lower its glycemic impact.

Citrus fruit – zest for life!

Lemons, oranges, grapefruit, limes and tangerines take pride of place in the Mediterranean anti-cancer food basket. Studies suggest that citrus consumption may lower the risk of certain cancers, especially those along the digestive tract. This may be due to a variety of protective factors in the juice and peel of citrus fruits (d-limonene in lemon zest, tangeritin and nobiletin in tangerine peel, hesperidin in membranes) that are thought to help remove potentially carcinogenic substances from the body and inhibit cancer cell growth.

It's a good habit to always stock a basic supply of citrus fruit – especially lemons and limes – whose zest imparts a delicate, fresh flavor to dishes without any of the acidity that comes with using citrus juice. Zest can be grated into salad dressings, sauces, stews, used in fish dishes, desserts and baking. When eating citrus zest, use only untreated fruit as conventionally grown fruit is usually treated with toxic chemicals that protect it from insect and fungal attack.

Citrus peel and juice added to green or white tea and herbal infusions add refreshing flavors to these beverages. Lemon zest can be grated into plain yogurt or muesli for a tangy breakfast dish. Lemon juice drizzled over steamed vegetables, perhaps with a tablespoon of olive oil, brings them to life.

Raw or cooked?

While a purely raw-food diet may suit some individuals, most people benefit from eating both raw and cooked foods. Cooking softens harsh plant fibers, making it easier for our jaws, teeth and digestive systems to break down food without expending too much energy. Heat also reduces the risk of bacterial contamination. All this is particularly important for people whose digestive and immune systems are weakened by sickness or medical treatments.

Cooking also helps to break down potentially unhealthy substances in natural plant foods, such as oxalic acid in spinach or Swiss chard. Moreover, while some vitamins and enzymes do get destroyed during cooking, lightly cooked vegetables actually provide more nutrients than when they are eaten raw.

Take carrots. Because cooking breaks down their tough cell walls, lightly steamed carrots provide one-third more beta carotene than raw ones[29]. The same applies to other vegetables such as spinach, mushrooms, asparagus, cabbage and bell peppers. Cooking techniques matter too: according to a recent study, boiling and steaming carrots, zucchini and broccoli better preserves antioxidants than sautéing[30].

Another nutrient that becomes more available through cooking is lycopene, an antioxidant found predominantly in the skins of tomatoes. It has been linked to a lower incidence of cancer, especially of the prostate. Cooking lycopene-rich foods boosts the availability of this precious nutrient: in whole tomatoes cooked for ½ hour at 190°F (88°C), lycopene levels are 35% higher than in raw tomatoes[31]. Tomato paste, made of cooked and pureed whole tomatoes, is a particularly concentrated source of lycopene. Not surprisingly, a study of people following a strict raw-food diet showed that they had low levels of lycopene[32].

Must we eat them every day?

No doubt about it, vegetables and fruits should be eaten daily, ideally at every meal and snack. They are the best source of water-soluble vitamins (vitamin C and all the B-vitamins), which are essential to a healthy immune system. Unlike fat-soluble vitamins, which our bodies can store, water-soluble ones get excreted when our bodies are not using them and so they need to be replenished constantly.

When spreading out our fruit and vegetable intake over the day, it's amazing how easy it is to get all the portions we need – and then some! Here's how:

- **Breakfast**: a bowl of Bircher muesli (p. 238) containing a grated apple and a generous handful of berries (2 portions of fruit).
- **Mid-morning snack**: a raw carrot (1 vegetable portion) dipped in Hummus (p. 199).
- **Lunch**: Greek salad with feta cheese or cubed chicken breast (p. 127) containing one tomato (1 vegetable portion), 1 serving of lettuce (1 vegetable portion), and some cubed cucumber and raw onion (1 more portion).
- **Afternoon snack**: A "Berry Booster" raspberry smoothie (p. 237) (1 portion fruit), an apple, pear, orange or tangerine (1 portion fruit) with a handful of almonds.
- **Dinner**: a serving of Lentil salad (p. 187) (1 vegetable portion) and 2 tablespoons of Garlicky spinach (p. 220) to accompany fish or chicken in Basic tomato sauce (p. 226, 1 vegetable portion).

Before we know it, we've eaten three portions of fruit and seven vegetable portions! Not so hard, is it? And tasty too!

The trick is to be on the look-out for ways to include vegetables and fruits at every possible opportunity. If we don't do this, it is easy for bread, pasta, pizza, cakes, cookies and candy bars – tasty and filling, but not nutritious – to creep in and displace the nutritious plant foods our bodies crave. This is why we should actively and intentionally seek these out, all day, every day. Once this becomes a habit, it gets increasingly easy.

Color me healthy

One way to remember to eat a wide variety of fruits and vegetables is to vary the colors of the plant foods we eat as much as possible. Different plant chemicals give fruits and vegetables their colors, and so the more colors we eat, the broader our plant nutrient intake will be.

The table on the next page shows the seven main color groups of foods. Eating one vegetable or fruit from each color group daily could be one way of ensuring that we are getting enough and keeping our diet varied so it doesn't become boring.

Frozen versus fresh?

Some vegetables and fruits – like peas or berries – have such short growing seasons that if we were to rely on eating them fresh we'd miss out. Frozen fruits and vegetables can prolong the seasons to provide a wide range of precious nutrients all year round. Although it may not taste quite like perfectly fresh vegetables, frozen produce is a nutritious and practical fall-back option for days when our fresh supplies are low and we have no time to go shopping.

Frozen vegetables and fruits have other advantages: they are cleaned and ready for use, cutting down on preparation time. This also means that when you are buying frozen vegetables, you are only paying for the edible portion and not for a pile of leaves that you will throw away.

If harvested, frozen and stored under optimal conditions, frozen produce offers a similar nutritional profile to fresh since it is usually picked at peak ripeness and frozen immediately after harvesting. Nonetheless, even frozen foods shouldn't be stored for more than 2-3 months at most as their nutritional value reduces with time. (This also applies to frozen fish or meat.)

The seven colors of health [33]

Colour and active phytonutrient	Food sources	Physiological functions
Red (lycopene)	Tomatoes, pink grapefruit, water melon; processed tomatoes (tomato paste, ketchup, soup, juice).	Antioxidant, induces enzymes that protect cells against carcinogens; may protect against prostate and lung cancers.
Red/Purple (anthocyanidins, proanthocyanidins, ellagic acid)	Red apples, red peppers, blackberries, blueberries, red cabbage, cherries, cranberries or cranberry juice/sauce, eggplant, red grapes or juice, red pears, plums, pomegranates, prunes, strawberries, red wine.	Antioxidant, anti-angiogenic, may help prevent the binding of carcinogens to DNA; may protect against gastro-intestinal cancers.
Orange (alpha and beta carotenes)	Carrots, mangos, apricots, cantaloupes, pumpkin, acorn squash, winter squash, sweet potatoes.	Antioxidant, may improve communication between cells; may help prevent lung cancer.
Orange/yellow (beta-cryptothanxin, a minor carotenoid)	Orange juice, oranges, tangerines, peaches, papayas, nectarines.	Antioxidant, may inhibit cholesterol synthesis needed to activate cancer cell growth.
Yellow/green (carotenoids lutein, zeaxanthin)	Avocados, peppers (green or yellow), collard greens, sweetcorn, cucumber, green beans, honeydew melon, kiwifruit, mustard greens, peas, green romaine lettuce, spinach, turnip greens, zucchini (with skin).	Help correct DNA imbalances; help stimulate enzymes that break down carcinogens.
Green (sulforaphane, isothiocyanate, indoles)	Broccoli, Brussels sprouts, bok choy, cabbage, cauliflower, kale, Swiss chard, watercress.	Stimulate the release of enzymes that break down cancer-causing chemicals in the liver; may inhibit early tumor growth.
White/green (allicin from the onion family ; flavonoids quercetin and kaempferol)	Garlic, onion, leek, celery, pears, endive, chives, arti-chokes, asparagus, mush-rooms.	Antioxidant, anti-tumor.

Don't worry too much about portion sizes; they are an approximate guideline and vary according to the density of the food in question. Here are rough guidelines[34]:

Quick guide to vegetable portions
(Each item represents one portion)

- **Green leafy vegetables:** 2 broccoli spears, 8 small cauliflower florets, 4 heaped tablespoons each of kale, spring greens or green beans.
- **Cooked vegetables:** 3 heaped tablespoons of cooked vegetables such as carrots, peas, spinach, or chard. Frozen vegetables: roughly the same quantity as you would eat as a fresh portion.
- **Salad vegetables:** 3 ribs celery, 2 inch piece of cucumber, 1 medium tomato, 7 cherry tomatoes.
- **Legumes:** 3 heaped tablespoons white beans, kidney beans, garbanzos, butter beans or lentils. Legumes only count as one daily portion, no matter how much you eat.

Quick guide to fruit portions
(Each item represents one portion)

- **Fresh fruit**
  Small: 2 plums, 2 mandarins, 3 apricots, 2 kiwi fruit, 7 strawberries, 14 cherries, 6 lychees
  Medium: 1 medium-sized apple, banana, pear, orange, nectarine, or 1 persimmon (also known as kaki or Sharon fruit)
  Large: half a grapefruit, 1 slice of papaya, 1 slice of melon, 1 large slice of pineapple, 2 slices of mango

- **Preserved fruit from a jar:** Roughly the same quantity of fruit that you would eat as a fresh portion: 2 pear or peach halves, 6 apricot halves, 8 segments of grapefruit. Eat this only if fresh fruit is not available and choose fruit preserved in fruit juice rather than in sugar syrup.

- **Juice:** A small glass (5 fl oz/150ml) of 100% freshly pressed fruit/vegetable juice or smoothie counts as a portion, but you can only count juice as one portion per day no matter how much you drink. This is because it contains very little fiber and is a more concentrated source of sugar than whole fruit.

It is best to buy from frozen-food specialists who process vegetables and fruits under optimal conditions and have rapid turnover. Check "best before" dates when selecting frozen foods and make sure they stay frozen on the way from the shop to your freezer. Lastly, frozen vegetables need less cooking time than fresh ones as they are usually blanched in hot water before being frozen.

Stick to vegetables and fruits, fish or meat that have been frozen without the addition of other ingredients. Some frozen vegetables come with seasonings and sauces containing unhealthy fats, chemical additives, flavor enhancers, sugar or excess salt, so check labels carefully.

Should we go organic?

More and more people worried about pesticide residues in conventionally farmed produce are switching to organic food. Others believe that organically grown food contains more nutrients. The nutritional benefits of organic food are difficult to assess; indeed, while some studies indicate that organic foods contain greater concentrations of vitamins, minerals and healthy plant compounds, others do not back these up.

Organic food is not a viable option for everyone; some people do not live near a health-food shop and have no organic delivery scheme in their neighborhood. Others cannot afford organic food, which, because it is produced at a greater investment of labor, generally costs more than mass-produced food.

In a perfect world, none of our food would contain agricultural chemicals. However, as long as these are below officially permitted thresholds, the benefits of eating a wide variety of fresh vegetables outweigh the potential risks of chemical residues.

Nonetheless, people wishing to reduce potential exposure can do so by carefully choosing the types of non-organic fruit and vegetables they buy. One way to select healthy non-organic foods is to buy items from the Environmental Working Group's "least-contaminated" list, and to buy organically grown versions only of the foods on the "most-contaminated" list (Chapter 3, p. 48).

Incidentally, non-organic farmers who work on a small scale often use fewer agricultural chemicals than managers of larger, intensive farms; if in doubt, just ask at your local farm store whether and how their vegetables and fruits were treated.

If you eat conventionally grown food and are concerned about possible pesticide residues, these can be removed by peeling or thorough cleaning with a brush or a cloth under running water. When preparing leafy vegetables, such as cabbage or lettuce, the outer leaves should be removed and the rest washed thoroughly in fresh water. Some people wash fruits and vegetables in a basin of water with an added dash of detergent to remove fat-soluble pesticides that running water may not eliminate. If doing this, be sure to rinse off the soap thoroughly.

One more thing on organics: just because something is produced organically does not necessarily mean it is healthy. Thus, organic sugar, white bread or rice crackers will still be high in calories, provide few nutrients and raise blood glucose. Likewise, the fact that an animal has been reared organically does not necessarily mean that its meat or eggs will contain more nutrients or a healthy omega-6-to-3 ratio, especially if it was confined to a small enclosure and fed grains high in omega-6 fatty acids, such as corn. So when choosing animal products, it's useful to find out how they were produced, for example by looking out for labels stating that the animals were grass-fed or consumed flax seeds.

The spice of life: anti-cancer herbs and spices

One of the salient characteristics of the Mediterranean diet is its liberal use of herbs and spices. Historically, these were used for food preservation and medicinal purposes, rather than purely as flavorings to tickle our taste buds. Our ancestors knew that many herbs and spices had anti-microbial and anti-fungal properties. They are now known also to have a wide range of antioxidant, anti-inflammatory, cancer cell growth-inhibiting and detoxifying actions[35]. Moreover, by adding complex aromas to dishes, herbs and spices allow us to cut back on our use of salt.

> ## Selecting and storing herbs and spices
>
> - To enjoy the freshest herbs, grow your own: even a window box can accommodate a small selection of herbs such as thyme, parsley, chives or savory.
> - To store fresh herbs, rinse, shake them dry and refrigerate in a sealable plastic tub lined with kitchen paper; this will keep them fresh for up to a week. When buying or harvesting more herbs than you need, wash, dry, chop and freeze them in small containers. (Label these – frozen herbs all look alike!)
> - Dried herbs and spices should be bought in small quantities and used up as quickly as possible; there is little point in trying to save money by buying large "value-packs" which will decline in nutritional quality and flavor after a few months. They should be stored in dry, dark, cool surroundings with their lids tightly sealed.

For instance, labiates, the family of leafy herbs that include mint, thyme, marjoram, oregano, basil and rosemary, contain essential oils with anti-inflammatory properties called terpenoids; they are thought to encourage cancer cells to self-destruct and may reinforce conventional cancer treatments.

Apiums, the group of herbs that includes parsley, celery and celeriac, contain antioxidant compounds such as apigenin whose anti-tumor properties have been shown in laboratory studies to inhibit angiogenesis, the growth of blood vessels that supply tumors with nutrients[36].

Other herbs and spices with anti-cancer properties include capsaicin (in cayenne and red chili peppers), fennel, fenugreek, ginger, rosemary and black cumin[37], cinnamon, coriander, cumin, bay leaf, sage and black pepper.

Most fresh herbs are delicate and lose their flavor and color if cooked for too long; it is best, therefore, to add them to dishes towards the end of cooking. Most dried herbs, on the other hand, unfold nicely during cooking so it's fine to add them early on.

Dried spices are generally "awakened" by cooking and need some time in a hot, damp environment before developing their full aroma. Toasting whole spices before grinding them – a common practice in Indian cooking – intensifies their flavors. To toast, heat a pan over moderate heat, add whole spices and shake until a warm, nutty aroma arises after about 30 seconds; pound with a mortar and pestle and return to pan.

Tumor-inhibiting terpenoids[38]

Terpenoid	Herbs that contain the active terpenoid
Carvone	Caraway, spearmint and dill
Cineole	Coriander, lavender, rosemary, sage and thyme
Farnesol	Lemongrass, chamomile and lavender
Geraniol	Lemongrass, coriander, melissa, basil and rosemary
Limonene	Caraway, mints, cardamom, dill, celery seed, coriander and fennel
Menthol	Peppermint
Perillyl alcohol	Lavender, spearmint and sage
a-Pinene	Caraway, coriander, fennel, juniper berry, rosemary and thyme

Cooking ground spices in oil before adding other ingredients also releases their flavors.

When it comes with cooking with herbs and spices, let's allow our imagination and our taste buds to be our guides. The Mediterranean cuisine is remarkably inclusive and accommodates a wide range of flavors.

Golden goodness: turmeric

Turmeric, and more particularly curcumin, the compound that gives it its golden color, has been used by Indian Ayurvedic doctors for thousands of years to treat a wide variety of ailments. It is thought to reduce inflammation, inhibit the rapid growth of cancer cells, induce their self-destruction and discourage the growth of blood vessels feeding tumors. Cell culture, animal studies and some human trials have suggested therapeutic or preventive effects associated with curcumin; more trials are underway to confirm these effects in humans.

Curcumin is not easily absorbed, though its uptake may be enhanced if it is eaten with black pepper[39] or cruciferous vegetables[40]. Onions and curcumin consumed together may also offer added protection, one study showed: After patients with pre-cancerous colonic polyps took daily quercetin and curcumin supplements for six months, more than half their polyps disappeared and the remaining ones shrank by half.[41]

Fresh turmeric (resembling ginger roots, only smaller), available from health-food shops, is more fragrant than the powder. Two grated teaspoons of the fresh rhizome are roughly equal to one teaspoon of the powder. (Caution: fresh turmeric stains skin and clothes, so wear rubber gloves when handling it.) Store fresh turmeric in an airtight container in the refrigerator and the powdered spice in a sealed container in a cool, dark place. It's best to eat pure turmeric rather than curry powder as commercial curry blends contain only very small amounts of curcumin.

Turmeric goes well with any dish involving onions, ginger and garlic, such as North African, Indian or Asian dishes, but it also works well in recipes where it would not be traditionally found — for instance, dishes involving mustard (e.g. Mackerel with mustard, p. 173, or Tofu Dijonnaise, p. 196). Egg salad's golden hue is enhanced by the addition of turmeric, as are pie crusts and breads, or rice, quinoa and pasta when turmeric is added to their cooking water.

Beans — vegetables or starch?

A valuable plant food with many health benefits, beans have been cultivated and consumed for thousands of years around the Mediterranean. Because beans, lentils and garbanzos — also called legumes — come out of pods that grow on bushes, they are widely considered vegetables. However, their unique nutrient make-up – they are rich both in carbohydrates and protein – puts them in a separate category.

Beans contain several types of plant chemicals that may play a role in cancer prevention, such as saponins, protease inhibitors and phytic acid. Many legumes also contain natural compounds that resemble a weak form of estrogen. These may protect against certain types of cancer – notably breast and prostate cancer[42].

Phytoestrogens: soy, flax and co.

Phytoestrogens are plant chemicals that resemble estrogens – sex hormones produced by our bodies. They are found in many foods; soy has the highest concentration. Opinions diverge over the benefits of eating soy for cancer prevention. Some say that phytoestrogens, and particularly the kind called isoflavones, may help prevent certain types of cancer, notably hormone-dependent cancers of the breast and prostate. Asian women are less prone to breast cancer than western women and some researchers think this is because they eat more soy[43].

However, conclusions from Asian studies do not necessarily apply to western populations: Asian women eat different types of soy foods, and from an earlier age, than western women. In Japan or China, commonly eaten soy products include tofu, soy beans and soy milk as well as fermented soy foods such as tempeh, miso and natto. These are less popular in the west, where most dietary isoflavones are derived from highly processed soy flour and protein commonly added as extenders and fillers in industrial baking and canning.

There is also some disagreement over whether soy is safe for breast-cancer survivors, amid concerns that phytoestrogens may promote cancer recurrence. A team of researchers analyzing data from the large-scale Shanghai Breast Cancer Survival Study recently found that those women eating the most soy protein – up to 11 grams a day – had a 32% lower risk of breast cancer recurrence compared to those with the lowest intake of soy protein[44]. However, until more evidence is available, people who have had hormone-dependent cancers should consume soy in moderation.

When you eat soy foods, choose relatively unprocessed ones such as plain tofu or tempeh and unsweetened, unflavored soy milk and yogurt. Avoid highly processed burgers, patties or sausages made with soy that are designed to mimic the taste of meat. Also avoid soy isoflavone supplements because they often contain excessive amounts of phytoestrogens.

People who do not like soy or are allergic to it can obtain phytoestrogens from other plant compounds called lignans. Lignans, which also have antioxidant properties, are converted by our gut bacteria into estrogenlike molecules, though they are not as similar to our bodies' own estrogen as are the isoflavones in soy. Flax seeds are a rich source of lignans, but they are also found in lower concentrations in sesame seeds, whole rye, wheat, oats and barley, legumes and many fruits, berries and vegetables.

A recent human intervention study indicated that flax seeds may protect against prostate cancer: men with prostate cancer who ate 30 grams (three tablespoons) of ground flaxseed each day for one month had decreased cancer cell proliferation compared to similar men who did not eat flaxseed.[44a]

Flax seed is a minor dietary component in most countries, but it is useful to eat it regularly, not only for its lignan content but also for the omega-3 fats and fiber it provides. To make full use of flax seeds' health virtues they should be ground into a fine powder (an electric coffee grinder works well for this); this allows our body to absorb two to four times more of their nutrients than eating them whole[45]. Once they are ground they should be refrigerated. It's fine to bake with ground flax seeds at moderate temperatures; neither the fats nor the lignans in flax are significantly affected by baking and cooking[46].

Because they are high in fiber and protein, beans promote a feeling of satiety by slowing down digestion. Moreover, despite their high starch content, beans are generally low-glycemic foods (see GI/GL table on pp. 42-43), thus keeping blood glucose levels balanced. Dark-skinned legumes, such as black or red beans, also contain antioxidant compounds called anthocyanidins.

Beans and lentils are not only healthy, they're also inexpensive, versatile and easily integrated into many recipes. They enhance the flavor of meat when combined in stews (as, for example, in the Moroccan chicken and garbanzo soup on p. 142) and because they taste bland, they are an excellent vehicle for other strong flavors such as tomato, garlic, olive oil, ginger and fresh herbs.

Silencing the "musical fruit"

What puts many people off eating legumes is that they can cause embarrassing intestinal gas. When carbohydrates in beans, called oligosaccharides, are digested by bacteria in the gut this produces gas. In many cuisines beans are cooked with aniseed, fennel or coriander seeds, savory, cumin, caraway and turmeric to reduce this reaction. Infusions of fennel, aniseed, peppermint, coriander or chamomile sipped during or after the meal may also help.

Soaking beans for 12-24 hours, rinsing them thoroughly after soaking and cooking them until they are soft may also reduce oligosaccharides. In Asia a type of seaweed, kombu, is added to beans as they cook to speed up cooking and reduce oligosaccharide levels. Kombu can be obtained in most health food stores. Adding vinegar after cooking may render legumes more digestible, too. Anecdotal evidence suggests that lentils and garbanzos may be less "gassy" than other dried beans.

Sprouting legumes before cooking them may also help make them more digestible. Sprouting breaks down the starch portion of beans into simpler, easier-to-digest carbohydrates and also increases protein, vitamin and enzyme content. To sprout beans and grains, soak them overnight, drain, rinse and leave them in a strainer in a semi-dark but well ventilated place for 1-3 days, rinsing daily until tiny sprouts start to appear.

Lastly, thorough chewing is important; taking small mouthfuls and chewing each one 30-40 times helps pre-digest the beans, leaving less work for the bacteria to do later. Think Mediterranean: taking time to savor every mouthful makes the food we eat easier to digest and absorb.

Whole grains: enjoy in moderation

When left in full possession of their germ and bran, where all the vitamins, minerals, fats and fiber are concentrated, whole grains can be a good source of nutrients. They contain antioxidant vitamin E, most B vitamins and the minerals magnesium and zinc, as well as plant chemicals thought to have anti-cancer properties, such as saponins and lignans.

Much of this goes missing when grains are processed, so the grains we eat should be in their whole and most natural state. However, even whole grains aren't as nutritious as is widely thought. When comparing the nutrient density of various foods, researchers found that wholegrain bread was at best moderately nutritious. Vegetables and fruits such as spinach, broccoli, tomatoes, strawberries and blueberries have a considerably higher nutrient content than whole wheat bread and contain significantly fewer calories[47].

According to Colorado State University Professor Loren Cordain, a specialist in pre-agrarian human nutrition, "on a calorie-by-calorie basis whole grains are lousy sources of fiber, minerals, and B vitamins when compared to fresh fruit and veggies, lean meats and seafood."[48] He notes that a 1,000-calorie (4,186 kj) serving of fresh fruits and vegetables has between two and seven times as much fiber as a comparable serving of whole grains. In fruits and vegetables most of the fiber is the soluble kind that is gentle on the intestines – unlike the harsh insoluble fiber of most whole grains.

Whole grains' mineral status is even poorer: according to Professor Cordain, a 1,000-calorie serving of whole grain cereal contains 15 times less calcium, three times less magnesium, 12 times less potassium, six times less iron and two times less copper than a comparable serving of fresh vegetables.

Not only do grains contain fewer nutrients than some vegetables and fruits; some wholegrain products can be difficult to digest and assimilate. Fermentation (for instance by using sourdough), sprouting, soaking and cooking can help; this is how grains were traditionally prepared in the Mediterranean region.

So why not try eating gruels of grains or flakes that have been soaked overnight and slowly cooked in the morning, rather than factory-made bread or dry flakes out of a box? (See recipes for Bircher muesli, p. 238 or Hazelnut-chocolate porridge, p. 242.)

Watch your wheat

People diagnosed with a condition called celiac disease have a severe reaction to gluten, a protein found in grains like wheat and rye. Unless they avoid grains (and a wide range of processed meals, sauces, candy and snacks) containing gluten, they have a heightened risk of developing cancers of the small intestine[49]. In others, wheat may provoke allergic symptoms such as skin rash, bloating or nausea, which disappear when wheat is cut out of the diet.

The ubiquitous nature of wheat – it's in most processed foods from breads, cereals and cookies to sauces, dressings and snacks – means that many of us get heavily exposed to it. For this reason, it's useful to rotate different grains, and to replace at least some of the wheat we eat with grains containing less gluten, such as barley, spelt or oats, as well as with gluten-free grains like buckwheat, rice, amaranth, millet or quinoa.

Many people eat grains five or six times a day (or more!): toast or cereal at breakfast; cookies throughout the morning; a sandwich or pasta for lunch; a candy bar or cup cake in the afternoon and pizza for dinner. Eating this many grain products crowds out more nutritious vegetables and fruits. So while many of us don't need to give up grains entirely, we might consider reducing our cereal intake and replacing at least some of it with vegetables and fruit, nuts and seeds.

Starchy carbohydrates: friend or foe?

We don't need to cut all sweet or starchy foods out of our diets, but it's useful to choose carbohydrates that help us maintain balanced blood glucose and insulin levels. Here's how we can limit the glycemic impact of carbohydrates and balance blood-glucose levels.

- *The GI/GL of a carbohydrate can be reduced if it is eaten together with **protein or fat**; these slow down the speed at which the stomach empties. Thus, a plate of pasta with tomato sauce will cause a stronger blood-sugar increase than the pasta served with tomato sauce containing lean meat, fish or tofu, drizzled with a teaspoon of olive oil and sprinkled with parmesan cheese.*
- ***Acids** such as lemon juice and vinegar added to a meal can reduce its glycemic effect; in one study, vinegar lowered the GI of a starchy meal from 100 to 64[50].*
- ***Fermentation** can lower the glycemic impact of a food; thus, traditional sourdough bread has a lower GI than bread made with industrial yeast. In one study, the GI of sourdough bread was 68, compared 100 for non-sourdough bread [51].*
- *The **ripeness** of a food can also affect its glycemic impact; the riper a fruit or vegetable, the more sugars it often contains and the higher its GI ranking. The GI of bananas, for instance, ranges from 30 in under-ripe fruit to 70 in their over-ripe brothers[52].*
- ***Fiber** content also has a bearing on a food's GI value. Soluble fiber – prevalent in apples, oats and legumes – slows down the release of carbohydrates into the blood stream. Insoluble fiber, such as wheat bran, on the other hand, has little protective effect: when whole grains are finely milled, they are digested and absorbed almost as quickly as refined grains.*
- ***Different types of starch** have different GI values; some convert more quickly into blood sugar than others. Thus, potatoes – especially when mashed (GI of around 80) or baked in the oven (GI in the low 90s) convert more quickly into blood sugar than, say, sweet potato (GI in the 50s) because of the different types of starch they contain. Most kinds of rice are quickly converted into blood sugar; their GIs range from the mid-50s to the mid-80s (see p. 42). Hulled barley, cooked and eaten just like rice, contains different starches and accordingly is broken down more slowly; it has a GI of 22. Replace rice with barley wherever possible.*
- *Certain **foods and spices** eaten with higher-GI carbohydrates can dampen their glycemic impact; these include onions and garlic, blueberries, cherries, raspberries and cinnamon.*

Pulling the sweet tooth

Humans are programmed to seek out sweetness. The first food we taste as soon as we're born is sweet: our mothers' milk. Throughout evolution, we learned that sweet foods are rarely, if ever, poisonous and came to appreciate the burst of energy that follows the consumption of a sweet food. In nature, optimum ripeness and nutrient content of a fruit or vegetable is often signaled by its sweetness, a fact that can't have escaped our ancestors.

For all these reasons, sugary and sweet tastes have always appealed to the human palate. As long as sugar was rare – Paleolithic man ate at most two kilos per year, in the form of painfully obtained wild honey – our love of sweet foods didn't represent much of a health risk. However, now that sugar and sweeteners are over-abundant and cheap we can indulge our sweet cravings to our heart's content, with devastating health consequences. Remember, the average American now consumes about 155 pounds of sugar per year - a staggering three pounds each week!

Which sugars should we eat?

There's no easy answer, but there's an honest one: no sugar is truly healthy. Until about 100 years ago humans did not eat concentrated sugars several times a day, and our organisms aren't well equipped to deal with this. However, some sweeteners are less damaging than others. Here are some suggestions for the least unhealthy way of adding sweetness to our food.

- *Wean yourself off sugar gradually: keep a food diary to track which sweet foods you eat, how much and how often. Next, slowly reduce the amount of sugar you put in drinks, the number of sodas you drink or the number of sweet snacks you eat. For example, over four weeks you can reduce the number of sugars in your coffee from three, to two, to one, to none. Train yourself to eat dark chocolate, starting with 60% cocoa content, then 65%, next 75%, then 85% and so on. After a while, the sugary foods you used to love will taste cloyingly sweet.*

- *Sugar masks flavor and so, as you reduce your sugar intake, your taste buds will become increasingly sensitive to the satisfying flavor of naturally sweet food. After several weeks of conscious low-sugar eating, an apple or a pear can taste like the sweetest, most succulent treat on earth! Vegetables, too, can taste sweet – for example slow-roasted bell peppers or slowly caramelized onions, or pumpkin, peas, beets and carrots. For those who like crunchy snacks, raw nuts and seeds – almonds, cashews, pecans, walnuts or pumpkin seeds – may be a satisfying alternative to candy, though they should be eaten in moderation as they are rich in calories.*

- *Honey in moderation. The most natural source of sugar is honey. Our ancient ancestors used it not so much as a sweetener, but as convalescent food and medicine. This is not surprising: Honey has remarkable antioxidant, anti-microbial, tumor-killing and anti-inflammatory properties. Use raw honey that has not been heat-treated; the best place to find this is a health food shop or farmers' market. While most types of honey have high glycemic-index rankings, acacia honey — runny and delicately flavored — has a low GI of 32[53]. Acacia honey costs more than sugar, but since you'll be consuming very little (even honey is sugar, so eat it very sparingly), a little will go a long way!*

- **Use natural sweeteners in small quantities.** *In my recipes I used the least amount of sweetener I felt I could get away with. As you transition to low-sugar eating, adding an extra smidgen of honey to these recipes won't do much harm as the sugar content will still be well below that of most conventional recipes, not to mention shop-bought desserts, cakes and cookies.*

- **Other natural sugars,** *like dehydrated cane sugar or maple syrup, have GI ratings similar to those of table sugar. They are acceptable in moderation but have no therapeutic value.*

- **Agave syrup and xylitol** *are two fashionable sweeteners with very low GI values. Both are derived from plants, but, unlike honey, they undergo heavy processing. They have other drawbacks: agave syrup, for one, contains as much as 90% fructose, which contributes to weight gain, heart disease and intestinal problems if eaten in large quantities. Moreover, a recent study found that pancreatic cancer cell growth was fuelled just as readily by fructose as by glucose[54]. Xylitol, a sugar alcohol extracted from birch bark may cause bloating and can have a chemical aftertaste. In contrast to honey, neither of these sweeteners offers cancer-protective benefits; they are simply lower-glycemic alternatives to sugar.*

- **Eat desserts as an occasional treat only,** *for example two to three times a week. Try eating stewed fruit after a meal and snack on fruit, nuts and seeds. A square of dark chocolate (minimum 70% cocoa content) after a meal can be very satisfying.*

- **An effective strategy for preventing after-dinner sweet-snacking** *is to thoroughly brush, floss and rinse your teeth as soon as the meal is over. After all that time and effort spent on oral hygiene, you won't want to go through it all again for the sake of a few sugary snacks, will you? (The minty taste in your mouth will put you off food anyway.)*

- **Getting enough sleep** *can help curb sugar cravings. When we feel fresh and rested in the morning, we are less likely to need to climb aboard the blood-sugar roller coaster (coffee, sweet pastries, sugary cereals, day-long snacking) than when we feel tired and irritable upon rising. Likewise, when we feel the urge to snack in the evening, maybe it's actually our body telling us to go to bed.*

The fats of life

Type of fat	Food source
Monounsaturated fat	Olive oil, rapeseed oil, peanut oil, avocados, nuts and seeds
Polyunsaturated fat (High in omega-3)	**Animal sources**: Fatty, cold-water fish (such as sardines, salmon, mackerel, anchovies, herring); eggs, milk and meat from farm animals fed omega-3 rich feed or from wild animals **Plant sources** : flaxseeds, walnuts, walnut oil, rapeseed oil, green leafy vegetables, purslane
Polyunsaturated fat (High in omega-6)	Most seed oils (safflower, sunflower, corn, soy, cottonseed), nuts and seeds
Saturated fat	Animal products (such as meat, poultry, seafood, eggs, dairy products, lard and butter), and coconut, palm and other tropical oils
Trans fat (AVOID!)	Partially hydrogenated vegetable oils, commercial baked goods (such as crackers, biscuits and cakes), fried foods (such as donuts and chips), vegetable shortening and margarine

Some facts about fats

To many people, the very notion of a "healthy fat" sounds like a contradiction in terms: decades of fat phobia have obscured the understanding that certain fats are crucial to a wide range of bodily functions, including immune health and hormone balance.

Fats should make up about a third of our daily calorie intake. Of this, roughly a third can come from saturated fats, another third from monounsaturated fats and the rest from polyunsaturated fats (see table above). Polyunsaturated fats are our main sources of omega-3 and omega-6 fatty acids, and as we saw in Chapter 3, they should be eaten in a healthy balance, with an omega-6-to-3 ratio of roughly 2:1 or 3:1.

Polyunsaturated fats are easily damaged when exposed to heat, light or oxygen as in cooking or processing. This causes free radicals to form which can trigger cancerous changes in cells. To prevent them from getting damaged (oxidized), cold-pressed, extra-virgin polyunsaturated oils should be stored in a dark, cool place and should not be used for cooking or sautéing.

These oils are best enjoyed in salad dressings, fruit and vegetable smoothies or drizzled over food just before serving. Indeed, this may boost the nutritional qualities of the greens you eat. In vegetables eaten with olive oil or butter, for example, certain nutrients – such as beta carotene or lycopene – are more easily absorbed[55-56]. As fat makes most vegetables taste better, it may also encourage vegetable skeptics – especially children – to eat their greens.

For cooking the best fats to use are olive oil (the most "Mediterranean" of fats), ghee (clarified butter) or coconut oil. Extra virgin olive oil contains antioxidant phenols and squalene that are thought to be cancer-protective[57]. However, these beneficial compounds may be destroyed by excess heat, so to make the most of olive oil's nutrients it's best to use as little as possible during cooking, and to drizzle a little more oil over the food as we eat it.

When cooking with olive oil, it should not be heated to the point at which it begins to smoke; if this happens, discard the oil and cool the pan down before starting anew. Different oils have different "smoke points" at which they start to degrade, creating free radicals. For extra virgin olive oil this is around 320°F (160°C); it can thus be used for cooking and baking at moderate temperatures.

Oils rich in omega-3 fats, such as flax, hemp or walnut oil, should not be heated. Even canola oil should be handled with care, for although it contains about 70% of stable monounsaturated fat and manufacturers recommend its use in cooking, it is also rich in omega-3 fats that degrade when heated. It's best to use this oil cold, like all extra-virgin, cold pressed polyunsaturated plant oils.

Fatty fish for optimal omegas

Oily fish, an integral part of the Mediterranean diet, provides two types of omega-3 fatty acids called EPA (eicosapentanoic acid) and DHA (docosahexanoic acid) that are vital to human health and are thought to have anti-cancer properties. Our body can synthesise EPA and DHA from plant sources of omega-3 fats such as flax or walnut oil, but this is a complex process requiring various nutrients and enzymes, and in many people the conversion is not very efficient. This is why fish oils are probably the most efficient way of obtaining omega-3 fats.

Omega-3 fatty acids in fish [58]

Type of fish	Amount of fish required (in grams) to provide approximately 1 g of EPA and DHA
Herring	
Pacific	45 g / 1.5 oz
Atlantic	60 g / 2 oz
Sardines	60 – 85 g / 2-3 oz
Mackerel	60 – 240 g / 2-8.5 oz
Salmon	
Atlantic, wild	60 – 100 g / 2-3.5 oz
Atlantic, farmed	45 – 70 g / 1.5-2.5 oz
Trout, rainbow	
Farmed	85 g / 3 oz
Wild	100 g / 3.5 oz
Tuna	
Tinned (white, canned in water)	110 g / 4 oz
Fresh	75 – 350 g / 2.5-12 oz
Halibut	85 – 210 g / 3-7.5 oz
Oyster	
Pacific	70 g / 2.5 oz
Farmed	225 g / 8 oz
Flounder/Sole	200 g / 7 oz
Shrimp (mixed species)	310 g / 11 oz
Clam	350 g / 12.5 oz
Cod	
Pacific	650 g / 23 oz
Atlantic	350 g / 12.5 oz
Haddock	425 g / 15 oz
Scallop	500 g / 17.5 oz

The intakes of fish given are very rough estimates because oil content may vary markedly with species, season, diet, and packaging and cooking methods.

Oily fish such as mackerel, sardines, salmon, trout, anchovies or herring are particularly rich in omega-3's and we should ideally eat these at least two times a week. The table on page 81 shows the omega-3 content of commonly eaten fish, indicating approximately how much fish we need to eat to obtain 1g a day of DHA and EPA.

There are some caveats. For one, it's worth bearing in mind that the bigger fish, like tuna, shark or swordfish, may be contaminated by pollutants. As they are at the end of the marine food chain, they concentrate the pollutants present in the smaller fish they eat. It's better to eat smaller, less polluted fish; besides, they are also substantially cheaper. Furthermore, sardines, mackerel and herring are not threatened with extinction, unlike some larger fish; thus we can enjoy these regularly without guilt pangs.

Salmon has been the subject of much debate. While it is an excellent source of omega-3 fats, the more affordable farmed salmon has come under scrutiny in recent years because of its potential contamination by polychlorinated biphenyls (PCBs) and chlorinated pesticides[59]. Farmed salmon from northern Europe is among the worst affected and our best bet appears to be wild salmon.

The best and safest way to enjoy fish is to vary the types of fish you eat as much as possible. When eating salmon, remove the skin and visible fat since PCBs are stored in the fat portion. Canned salmon is also useful, since almost all cans are made from the least contaminated wild Pacific salmon.

As with all food, I believe it's best to eat fish fresh, rather than canned, for optimal nutritional value. However, because conserved fish is tasty and convenient, this is fine as long as you alternate fresh and canned fish. Most fish cans are lined with epoxy resins that might release trace amounts of bisphenol-A into the cans' contents. However some manufacturers have begun using BPA-free cans and this trend is set to increase.

Go nuts!

Nuts and seeds – very popular in all Mediterranean countries – and their "butters" (finely ground creamy pastes sold in health food shops) are another source of healthy fats and proteins. Most nuts contain a high proportion of stable monounsaturated fats and antioxidants such as beta carotene, vitamin E and other compounds that protect their fats from going rancid. Some – such as walnuts – are also rich in omega-3 fats.

The best way to ensure nuts' freshness is to crack them yourself. When you buy pre-cracked nuts, they should be fresh and be kept in a cool, dark place. Storing them in tightly closed containers in the refrigerator reduces the risk of their fats getting damaged. Nuts should not be toasted at high temperatures; any toasting should be done at moderate heat (in an oven no hotter than 210°F (100°C), not a skillet) and they should be eaten immediately. Avoid roasted nuts sold as snacks; not only are these often roasted at high temperatures, but they generally contain lots of salt.

The nuts most suitable for toasting are almonds, hazelnuts or pecans because they are high in monounsaturated fatty acids which are stable at higher temperatures. Walnuts, pumpkin seeds and flax seeds contain more of the fragile omega-3 fatty acids and are best eaten raw, or toasted at very moderate temperatures (around 170°F (80°C)). It's best to limit peanuts, which may contain carcinogenic compounds (aflatoxins) produced by certain fungi.

Cocoa and chocolate: healthiest treat in town

Because they are rich in antioxidants and are, for most people, a source of great pleasure, good-quality chocolate and cocoa occupy a privileged position in any healthy pantry. Cocoa contains antioxidant compounds called procyanidins that are also found in red wine; two to three squares of good-quality chocolate containing 70-85% cocoa solids are equivalent to a 125 milliliter glass of procyanidin-rich red wine [60].

Research into the link between cocoa and cancer is still in its infancy, but scientists have observed that cocoa procyanidins slow the development of breast cancer in laboratory cell cultures[61], prostate cancer in rats[62] and may lower inflammation in humans[63].

The most efficient way of getting cocoa procyanidins into our bloodstream is by drinking chocolate drinks made with pure cocoa (Cocoa concoctions p. 264). Not only are these lower in fat than chocolate bars, they are also more easily absorbed because, being mixed with water or milk they are already in solution [64]. It used to be thought that milk (in cocoa drinks or milk chocolate) blocks the absorption of cocoa procyanidins, but research now shows this is not so; it merely slows their uptake [65].

One culinary factor that does reduce procyanidins in cocoa is baking soda, widely used as a leavening agent. Researchers investigating the effect of leavening agents on cocoa polyphenols found that in chocolate cakes leavened with baking soda, the amount of procyanidins declined by 84%; the same recipe prepared with baking powder, on the other hand, showed no procyanidin loss at all [66].

Not only cocoa's polyphenols suffer when they come into contact with baking soda. Other foods, such as cranberries, grapes, raisins, blueberries, apples, nuts and cinnamon may also experience antioxidant losses when combined with baking soda in cakes and baked goods; thus it is best to use baking powder or beaten egg white – a traditional French technique – to aerate baked goods (see Queen of Sheba chocolate cake on p. 262).

Most supermarkets sell chocolate with 70% cocoa content or more; if yours doesn't, you can find it at a health-food store or online. Because some cocoa-producing countries allow the use on cocoa plants of pesticides banned in the US and Europe, it is preferable to buy cocoa products with an organic certification.

The power of protein

When people hear the word "protein" they think of meat – not exactly known as an anti-cancer food. However, protein is found in many foods, not just meat, and is an essential part of our diet.

Because our bodies are continually breaking down protein from tissues and rebuilding these, we need to include adequate protein in our diets every day, ideally several times a day. According to the World Health Organization (WHO), healthy adults should eat 0.8 grams of protein per day for every kilogram of body weight. Thus, a woman weighing 132 pounds (60 kilos) should eat about 1.7 ounces (48 grams) of protein daily. (This is not equivalent to eating 1.7 ounces (48 grams) of chicken or tofu. Whole foods contain other substances – such as water or fat – which increase their weight. Thus, 1.7 ounces (48 grams) of protein equates to just over 6 ounces (170 grams) of skinless chicken breast or just over a pound (450 grams) of firm tofu.)

Eating more than the WHO-recommended amount is neither necessary nor healthy unless you are pregnant, lactating or a high-performance athlete. Eating protein at every meal stabilizes blood sugar levels and energy and helps us feel sated after meals. Thus, eaten regularly and in moderation, protein can help prevent cravings for sweet or starchy foods between meals, thus helping to maintain healthy weight.

In addition to supplying the raw material for bones, skin, organs and muscles, protein is needed to produce key immune-system components such as white blood cells. Moreover, for people losing weight due to illness it is important to eat sufficient high-quality protein to maintain muscle mass and support the immune system.

Protein is made up of sub-particles called amino acids. Animal protein such as meat, fish, eggs and dairy provides the complete range of amino acids we need. Plant foods, on the other hand, often lack one or more essential amino acids, reducing their protein value. However, by eating a wide range of legumes and whole grains, vegetarians can obtain all essential amino acids.

When eating animal protein it's best to choose meat from traditionally reared and pastured livestock, small oily fish from unpolluted waters, and eggs and dairy products from free-range animals nourished with grass and a small proportion of healthy seeds (including flax) rather than corn.

According to the World Cancer Research Fund/American Institute for Cancer Research, red-meat consumption (beef, pork, lamb) should not surpass 1.7 pounds (750 grams) of raw meat, or just over a pound (500 grams) of cooked meat per week. Lean white meat (chicken, turkey, skinless duck, rabbit), fish and eggs are healthy alternatives to red meat. Plant protein sources include soy products such as tofu and tempeh, dried beans and legumes, nuts and seeds and whole grains such as quinoa.

The recipes in this book provide a wide range of protein sources. Many of the soups, salads and purees involve the use of beans and legumes. Eggs are employed abundantly as they are a high-quality, inexpensive source of protein, omega-3 fats (if the hens that laid them ate an omega-3-rich diet) and other essential nutrients. In some recipes I have replaced flour or cream with almonds, hazelnuts, cashews and other nuts or seeds, slightly boosting the protein value of the dish. All meat recipes are based on lean poultry, rabbit and oily fish. This is not to say that I oppose all consumption of red meat; high-quality beef, lamb or pork are fine in modest portions and carefully prepared.

Milk and dairy products: be selective

Dairy, a popular protein source for vegetarians, is a controversial topic in the cancer context. Detractors claim that growth factors, hormones, saturated fats and pesticide residues in milk increase cancer risks, whereas defenders argue that in particular calcium and vitamin D in cows' milk have a protective effect[67].

The WCRF/AICR in its Expert Report states that milk probably decreases the risk of colon cancer and possibly that of bladder cancer, but that diets high in calcium from milk and dairy products increase the risk of prostate cancer.

What is certain is that the dairy products we eat in the industrialized west are not what they were 100 or more years ago. As we saw in Chapter 3, milk from intensively reared cows is likely to have less healthy omega-6-to-3 ratios, lower concentrations of protective conjugated linoleic acid and reduced antioxidant levels than that of pastured cows. Moreover, modern dairy products are often heavily treated, involving techniques like ultra-high temperature processing, condensation and drying, all of which affect the composition of dairy products and the way our bodies utilize them.

Milk is not indispensible to human health; indeed, many populations (most Asians, 60-80% of Africans and up to 15% of northern Europeans[68]) do not consume milk at all because their bodies cannot produce the enzyme needed to digest it, and they are nonetheless healthy! Calcium can be obtained from many other sources: small fish eaten with their bones (e.g. whole canned sardines), meat (when rendered on the bone in stews and broths), green leafy vegetables, nuts and legumes.

When consuming dairy, however, why not take our cues from the Mediterraneans? Here, dairy is usually eaten in small portions – almost as a condiment rather than a major food group. Milk by the glass is rarely consumed, and the most popular dairy products include fermented curds and cheeses made from goats', ewes' and occasionally cows' milk (e.g. kefir, yogurt, halloumi and feta cheese). Thanks to the effects of bacterial fermentation, even people who cannot digest lactose generally tolerate yogurt and hard cheeses like Parmesan, which have low lactose concentrations[69]. These are the dairy products I use in this book.

When you do eat dairy products, seek out the highest quality possible, made with milk from pastured organic cows. Moreover, vary the sources of your dairy products and include goats' and ewes' dairy. Not only are these animals usually less intensively farmed; their milk also contains more calcium and protein than cows' milk, so a little goes a long way. (Per 100 grams, ewes' milk delivers 193 milligrams calcium and 6 grams protein; goats' milk contains 134 milligrams calcium and 3.6 grams protein, and cows' milk offers 119 milligrams calcium and 3.3 grams protein.[70])

Keeping hydrated

An adult eliminates about two to four pints (one to two liters) of moisture through urine, sweat and breathing every day. To replenish this, we need to obtain at least the same volume of liquid through food and drink. This is particularly important for cancer patients undergoing chemotherapy because a steady intake of water can help flush out the toxic by-products of their treatments.

Nowadays many people don't drink water. Instead, they consume sugary sodas, juices made from concentrates, sweetened milk or yogurt beverages marketed as health foods, and caffeinated drinks like coffee and tea. While these liquids may go some way towards meeting our hydration needs, they also contain sweeteners, colorings, flavorings, preservatives, caffeine and, in the case of many sparkling soft drinks, bone-weakening carbonic and phosphoric acids, not to mention small amounts of potentially cancer-causing bisphenol-A leached into the drink from soda cans' linings. Because many of these drinks are high in calories, they fill us up, making us less interested in eating healthy, natural food. Avoid them wherever possible.

Even freshly pressed fruit juice should be drunk in moderation – one glass per day at most. Vegetable juices are a better alternative, with perhaps a tablespoon of olive or walnut oil added to further lower their glycemic impact. Tomato juice is a fine choice: not only does it have a weak glycemic effect, it is also an excellent source of lycopene, especially with added olive oil to aid its absorption.

When it comes to fruit, it's best to drink smoothies (p. 237) made from whole fruits, rather than just their juice. These delicious, thick drinks supply fiber, protein and fat from added yogurt, nuts or seeds and offer hydration and nourishment in one. They are particularly useful for people experiencing digestive complaints as a result of cancer treatments. Similarly, soups – raw or cooked (pp. 136-152) – are a convenient, easy-to-digest and nourishing way of getting vegetables in liquid form; these, too, can contain protein and fat to provide extra nutritional value.

Our main beverage of choice should be water, flavored, perhaps, with lemon, lime, fresh ginger or mint, according to our mood. This can be complemented by herbal tea (all-natural, without added flavorings or colorings) and antioxidant-rich green or white tea. Occasional cups of organic coffee or black tea are fine.

Water safety, a thorny issue

There is much debate about water quality amid fears that tap water may contain harmful compounds like pesticide and fertilizer residues, and disinfectants that produce potentially toxic contaminants such as chlorinated organic compounds.

According to the WCRF/AICR, there is currently no epidemiological evidence that any of these substances, singly or in combination, as currently regulated and usually consumed in water, foods or other drinks, has any significant effect on any cancer[71]. However, amid widespread concern over environmental pollution, water quality remains an issue.

Bottled water is not necessarily the healthiest option. Laboratory tests conducted for the US Environmental Working Group (EWG) found that 10 popular brands of bottled water contained 38 chemical pollutants altogether, with an average of 8 contaminants in each brand. Four brands were also contaminated with bacteria[72].

Considering also that bottled water costs many times more than tap water and the disposal of plastic bottles represents a heavy environmental burden, this may not be our best source of hydration.

Unlike bottled-water companies, municipal tap-water suppliers are obliged to publish all their water quality tests. To find out about the quality of your water, contact your local water supplier and ask to read their annual tap-water quality report. If you use a private well, have it tested by a specialist laboratory.

For added protection, the EWG recommends filtering tap water. Carbon filters (pitcher or tap-mounted) are affordable and reduce many common water contaminants like lead and by-products of the disinfection process used to treat municipal tap water. The more expensive reverse osmosis filters can remove some contaminants that carbon filters can't, like arsenic and perchlorate. When using water filters it is important to change the filters in them as often as their manufacturers advise; old filters can harbor bacteria and let contaminants through.

Don't forget to stay hydrated when you're out and about. Rather than buying expensive and potentially contaminated bottled water, buy a stainless steel bottle and bring along your own filtered water. The up-front investment will be quickly recouped by the money you save on commercially bottled water.

Tea – elixir of life?

While most westerners drink black tea, the inhabitants of Japan, China and the north African rim of the Mediterranean prefer green and white tea. All three come from the same plant, but white tea is the least processed and provides the largest quantity of antioxidant compounds[73], notably a flavonoid by the tongue-twisting name of epigallocatechin-3-gallate (EGCG) believed to account for many of the health benefits linked to green tea.

The more widely studied green tea is thought to have cancer-protective effects, including inhibiting angiogenesis and triggering apoptosis of cancer cells[74]. It may also reinforce the effects of certain chemotherapeutic agents[75] while lessening their negative side-effects[76]. There are countless varieties of green tea, but those with the highest EGCG levels are the Japanese Sencha, Gyokuro and Matcha teas, followed by Chinese Yunnan and Yuzan teas[77].

Green or white tea contains about half the amount of caffeine as black tea; nonetheless, if you are sensitive to the stimulating effects of caffeine, you can drink decaffeinated green tea. Alas, this contains only a third of EGCG found in regular tea because much of it is removed during decaffeination[78]. To reduce caffeine but maintain optimal EGCG levels, infuse regular green tea for 1-2 minutes in hot water, pour off the liquid, add more hot water and steep again for about 8 minutes. This method removes most of the caffeine but leaves both aroma and EGCG levels largely intact.

It's best to buy loose tea in small quantities; these are generally better-quality and fresher than green tea in tea bags. To avoid getting leaves in your beverage when using loose tea, the tea can be placed in a cotton-mesh bag (available in health-food stores or specialist tea shops) which can be placed in a tea pot or cup and where the tea has ample room to infuse. These filters can be rinsed after use and used repeatedly.

Generally, about one teaspoon of green or white tea should be used per 5fl oz (150ml) of water. To obtain the optimum amount of EGCG, these teas should be brewed with less-than-boiling water (175-185°F / 79-85°C) and steep for 8-10 minutes.

It used to be thought that green tea has to be drunk soon after brewing to obtain maximum EGCG levels. However, adding lemon juice to green tea helps to stabilize EGCG levels, which means you can drink it hours later – chilled lemon tea is particularly tasty in hot weather – and still obtain good EGCG intake. Indeed, researchers at Purdue University recently discovered that adding lemon juice and a little sugar enhanced the body's uptake of EGCG's four-fold as compared with green tea drunk plain[79].

To vary green tea's flavor you can add a piece of lemon zest, a slice of ginger or sprig of mint. Adding unsweetened lemon, orange or other fruit juices also makes for a more interesting drink. For a warming winter concoction, you can brew green tea with hot milk and add Indian "chai" spices (cinnamon, ginger, allspice, cardamom, pepper) and a smidgen of honey. (See recipes on p. 265)

Wine: friend or foe?

For millennia, grapes and wine have played an important role in those parts of the Mediterranean where alcohol consumption is permitted.

Anglo-Saxon-style "binge drinking" of large amounts of alcohol such as beer is rare around the Mediterranean. Here, alcohol consumption is generally moderate and takes place around mealtimes. A traditional Mediterranean meal includes moderate amounts of wine, accompanied by water to prevent over-indulgence.

Amid conflicting advice many people are confused about the cancer risk inherent in alcohol consumption – does it cause cancer, or may it actually offer protection?

Red wine contains high levels of resveratrol. This biologically active plant chemical with antioxidant and anti-cancer properties has been shown to reduce tumor incidence and to calm inflammation in laboratory animals. Red wine also contains high levels of anthocyanidins and procyanidins, other plant compounds with anti-cancer effects.

However, the ethanol in alcoholic drinks contributes to several common cancers, including those of the breast, mouth and throat and esophagus; some research also links it to liver and bowel cancer. The risk of some alcohol-related cancers is even greater in smokers.

Therefore the WCRF/AICR recommends that if alcohol is consumed at all, it should be limited to two drinks a day for men and one for women. The WCRF/AICR defines "one drink" as half a pint/250ml of normal strength beer or cider; a small (1oz/25ml) measure of spirits, or one small (4fl oz/125ml) glass of wine.

People who do not currently drink alcohol certainly should not take up wine-drinking for cancer-prevention. However, the occasional glass of high-quality red wine, consumed along with meals containing other protective plant compounds and healthy fats, is acceptable. Pregnant women (or those planning to become pregnant), people with pancreatic or liver disease and women who have a family history of breast cancer are advised to abstain from alcohol. If you have any doubts or are taking medication, talk to your doctor about the effect red wine may have on your health.

Polyphenol power

Not all red wines are created equal: some contain more antioxidants than others, depending on the soil and climate in which the grapes grew. Wines grown in the south-west of France, for instance, are exceptionally rich in procyanidins.

According to Roger Corder, Professor of Experimental Therapeutics at the William Harvey Research Institute in London and author of The Wine Diet, *one of the best-known south-western French wines, called "Madiran", typically contains three to four times more protective procyanidins than procyanidin-rich Argentininan Cabernet Sauvignon. "One glass of this wine can provide more benefits than two bottles of most Australian wine, without the obvious danger of excessive alcohol consumption," Corder notes.*

Slowly sipping wine and letting it linger in the mouth – a practice that sits comfortably with Mediterranean traditions – not only limits the amount of wine we drink; it may also increase the effectiveness of resveratrol, which is best absorbed through the mucous membranes in the mouth.

"Resveratrol is largely inactivated by the gut or liver before it reaches the blood stream, where it exerts its effects," explains Stephen Taylor, professor of pharmacology at the University of Queensland, Australia. *"Thus, most of the resveratrol in imbibed red wine does not reach the circulation. Interestingly, absorption via the mucous membranes in the mouth can result in up to around 100 times the blood levels, if done slowly rather than simply gulping it down."*

For teetotalers who still want to obtain these beneficial plant chemicals, there are many tasty alternatives. Other polyphenol-rich foods include raw cocoa (that hasn't been "dutched"), apples (especially the Red Delicious, Granny Smith and Reinette varieties), crab apples, cranberries (fresh or dried), raspberries, pomegranates and their juice, persimmons (also known as kaki or sharon fruit), nuts (especially walnuts, but also almonds and hazelnuts eaten with their skins), cinnamon and tea. Meanwhile, grapes, grape juice and mulberries are good sources of resveratrol.

All together now!

If only there were a precise scientific formula prescribing the perfect cancer-prevention diet. However, despite growing understanding of the nutritional factors that increase or lower our cancer risks, there is still much we don't know about the role of individual foods and nutrients.

This need not worry us unduly. For as we have seen, it isn't so much individual nutrients, but rather, the complex interplay of many different foods and their components, that keeps us healthy. It's not just *quantity* (the amount of healthy foods we eat a day) and *quality* (the nutrient density and freshness of the food), but particularly *variety* that matters.

Several studies have shown that eating a wide array of healthy foods is a key factor in preventing cancer. A 10-year investigation in the Netherlands, for instance, revealed that participants who ate the widest variety of vegetables were 36% less likely to develop cancer than people eating the least variety[80]. The *quantity* of vegetables consumed was not related to cancer incidence, the study showed, indicating that a large *variety* of plant-based anti-cancer substances, rather than any single compound, may offer protection against cancer.

Other studies suggest that eating a wide variety of natural foods may protect us from a whole host of cancers, notably those of the mouth and pharynx[81], the stomach[82], the digestive tract (from the esophagus to the rectum)[83],[84] and from breast cancer[85]. Remember: we are only talking of a variety of *healthy* foods, not a variety of processed foods.

Overall mortality – that is, the risk of dying prematurely of any illness such as cardiovascular disease or cancer – is also markedly reduced by eating a wide variety of healthy foods. In one study[86], women eating 16-17 healthy foods every day were found to be 42% more likely to outlive those who ate eight or fewer healthy foods daily. ("Healthy foods" in this study were defined as fruits, vegetables, whole-grain breads, cereals, fish and low-fat dairy products; "less healthy" ones were defined as red and processed meats, refined carbohydrates and sugars, and foods high in saturated or trans-fats.)

Different foods and nutrients eaten together can reinforce each other's cancer-fighting effects, as mentioned in Chapter 2. For example, the antioxidant effect of lycopene, the carotene found particularly in tomatoes, is boosted by various foods. Thus, in rats, the combination of tomatoes and broccoli eaten together slowed tumor growth faster than either food eaten on its own[87].

Another study found that tea and lycopene consumed together might have greater prostate cancer-protective effects than either consumed alone[88]. And in Taiwan, researchers recently discovered that a combination of omega-3-rich fish oils and lycopene synergistically inhibited the growth of human colon cancer cells in test tubes[89].

Even people who are genetically predisposed to cancer appear to benefit from eating a wide variety of plant foods. At the University of Montreal, a team of scientists studied women who carry the BRCA1 and BRCA2 genes that are associated with a significantly elevated risk of breast cancer. They discovered that the greater the variety of fruits and vegetables these genetically "at-risk" women ate, the less risk they had of developing cancer. For those who consumed more than 23 different fruits and vegetables per week, the risk diminished by 73%[90]!

My conclusion is simple, yet it has complex implications: the best cancer-prevention diet is one that contains a wide variety of fresh, unprocessed, seasonal vegetables and fruits, healthy fats, legumes, grains, fish, meats, herbs and spices that synergistically reinforce each other in promoting our health. It's simple, because we all know what these foods look like and where to obtain them. Yet it's complex because many of us need to significantly change our eating habits to include these foods in our diets every day, three or more times a day. Hopefully, this book can help.

Do nutritional supplements cut cancer risk?

Some 50% of Americans and 35% of Britons regularly take supplements[91]. Many of us see supplements as a sort of top-up health insurance, a safety net for when we don't get around to eating well.

In terms of cancer prevention, however, supplementation offers few documented benefits and at worst may actually increase risks. That's why the WCRF/AICR concludes in its Expert Report: "For otherwise healthy people, inadequacy of intake of nutrients is best resolved by nutrient-dense diets and not by supplements."

To be sure, many nutrients offer cancer protection, but these should ideally come from whole foods, not pills. For instance, according to the WCRF/AICR, the mineral selenium (found in Brazil nuts, whole grains, fish, crustaceans and meat) probably protects against prostate cancer, calcium (from kale, spinach and other green, leafy vegetables, nuts and seeds, canned whole sardines, tofu and dairy products) is thought to act against colon cancer and vitamin E (from plant oils, seeds, nuts and whole grains, berries and green leafy vegetables) may cut prostate-cancer risk.

Granted, swallowing a pill takes less time than preparing a healthy meal. However, whole, fresh food is a lot tastier, and also contains a much more complex range of nutrients than supplements can provide. For optimal nutrition, the food we eat should be as fresh as possible (ideally, locally grown in rich, healthy soil and eaten as soon as possible after harvesting), highly varied and carefully prepared. Long-distance transportation, long-term storage and overcooking can significantly reduce nutrient levels in foods.

There are exceptions where supplements are advisable. In people who have marked nutrient deficiencies or heightened nutritional needs, or who have trouble eating, digesting and absorbing food, supplementation is important. People over 50 who have difficulty absorbing vitamin B12 should supplement this. Moreover, women planning to conceive should take folic acid. Vitamin D is recommended for people who are not exposed to sufficient sunlight or those (such as the elderly or people with darker skin) who do not synthesize adequate vitamin D from sunlight. However, I caution against self-administering supplements; if you think you need extra nutrients or have difficulty digesting and absorbing the nutrients in your food, consult a doctor or nutritionist.

When eating becomes a chore

Cancer and its treatments put many people off their food. This is understandable; not only do many cancer patients feel anxious or depressed — emotional states that can suppress our appetite — but many cancer therapies also trigger physiological problems that make eating and digesting difficult.

Chemotherapy or radiotherapy, for instance, can irritate the digestive tract from the mouth (soreness, metallic taste, sore throat, trouble swallowing) via the stomach (nausea, vomiting) to the intestines (bloating, constipation, diarrhea).

Fatigue also affects many people undergoing cancer treatment, making it difficult for them to obtain and prepare foods from scratch. Getting help with shopping and food preparation when you are undergoing active treatment can be very helpful.

During treatment, focus on eating whatever foods you can get down and keep down. These should ideally contain lots of nutrients, but if you crave the occasional comfort of a chocolate chip cookie, enjoy one and let it lift your spirits.

During active cancer treatment it is important to remain hydrated and consume enough nutrients to prevent weight loss and weakness. Some people find liquid or pureed foods – such as soups, smoothies, fresh vegetable and fruit juices or vegetable purees – easiest to eat and digest. Such foods fulfill the double function of hydration and optimum nutrition, and are generally quick and easy to prepare.

Food safety during cancer treatment

Clean, safe food is crucial for people undergoing cancer treatment as they are vulnerable to bacteria, viruses or other foreign substances that can crop up in food. If you are undergoing cancer treatment, or are cooking for someone who is, follow these simple guidelines:
- *Keep cold foods cold (below 40°F/4°C) and hot foods hot (above 180°F/80°C).*
- *Wash fruits and vegetables thoroughly under running water before use.*
- *Wash the tops of cans before opening.*
- *Do not taste food that looks or smells strange. Do not eat food whose expiry date has passed. Avoid loosely packaged "street food" whose freshness you are not certain of.*
- *Avoid raw fish, meat (especially poultry), eggs, dairy products and mayonnaise, which may be contaminated with bacteria. Cook these foods thoroughly.*
- *Wash hands thoroughly before and after handling food and before eating.*
- *Make sure all tools, cutting boards, cutlery and plates are cleaned thoroughly. Tea towels and dishcloths should be changed after every use.*

Tips for nausea, vomiting, sore mouth or throat:
- *Eat small, frequent meals, rather than fewer, larger meals.*
- *Sip liquids – mainly water and herbal teas – throughout the day between meals but avoid drinking at meal times, which can exacerbate nausea. If you feel very nauseous, sip them slowly in small spoonfuls.*
- *Ginger can help calm nausea; infuse coarsely chopped raw ginger in hot water and sip it lukewarm, at room temperature or chilled, perhaps flavored with lemon and a little honey.*

(Check with your doctor before using ginger.) Peppermint tea can also be stomach-soothing.

- *Eat under calm, relaxed conditions. Rest after meals, preferably in a sitting position.*
- *Eat slowly and chew your food thoroughly to make it easier to digest.*
- *If strong flavors or odors turn you off, eat bland foods such as lightly poached chicken breasts or white fish, plain brown rice or pasta and vegetables such as carrots, sweet potatoes, peas, green beans or zucchini.*
- *Some people undergoing cancer treatment develop an aversion to the taste of red meat; replace this with lean poultry, fish and eggs to ensure sufficient protein intake.*
- *Wear comfortable, loose-fitting clothing.*
- *Get fresh air in your lungs by keeping your home well-aired and taking gentle walks with deep breathing. Yoga breathing exercises may help.*
- *Avoid eating hard-to-digest foods (fatty, fried or spicy dishes, for example).*
- *In case of vomiting, make sure you get enough liquids in the form of water, herbal infusions or fruit and vegetable soups and smoothies. If vomiting lasts longer than ½ hour, call your doctor.*
- *If you have sore gums, apply honey and leave for several minutes before swallowing.*
- *If head and neck radiotherapy is making your throat feel sore, have some honey before and after your treatment. One study showed that people who slowly swallowed four teaspoons of honey 15 minutes before and after treatment experienced significantly reduced oral mucositis — severely sore throat — than those rinsing with a saline solution, and also lost less weight[92]. Honey has many applications in cancer care; applied topically, it can promote the healing of radiation burns, chemotherapy-induced skin problems and surgical wounds[93].*

Tips for people suffering from constipation:

- *Keep well-hydrated; six to eight glasses of water and herbal infusions throughout the day.*
- *Eat fiber-rich foods — especially fruits and vegetables — at every meal. Whole grains, nuts and seeds can help too, but avoid wheat bran as it is hard on the intestines. If you have trouble chewing try grating, pureeing or blending your food.*
- *Stewed prunes can help set things in motion.*
- *Ground flax seed in soups, smoothies, cereals or baked goods can help promote bowel motility.*
- *Get as much light exercise, such as walking or bicycling, as your health permits.*
- *Eat plain, live yogurt or kefir daily to help maintain a healthy gut flora.*

Tips for people suffering from diarrhea:

- *Again, drink plenty of liquids to prevent dehydration; sip about eight glasses of water and herbal infusions throughout the day.*
- *Consume plenty of liquids and foods containing potassium and sodium, such as vegetable broth,*

bananas, green leafy vegetables, mushrooms, celery, broccoli or squash.

- *Temporarily reduce your intake of high-fiber foods (fresh vegetables, fruit, whole grains) and opt for apple or quince purees, rice and rice water, pasta and white toast until the diarrhea has stopped. Then return to a more fiber-rich diet.*
- *Eat plain, live yogurt or kefir daily to help maintain a healthy gut flora; if you find this hard to keep down, ask your doctor to recommend a probiotic supplement.*
- *Avoid fatty foods or large amounts of protein in a single meal.*

Having discussed in some detail all the foods that can boost our health, let's take a closer look at how we can fit these into our busy day-to-day lives.

Chapter Five

Let's Get Cooking!

Hopefully by now you're itching to rush out to the shops for a basket full of fresh produce, throw on your apron and rustle up a tasty Mediterranean meal.

More realistically, you're probably wondering where to start.

Unlike our great-grandmothers, most of us were never taught to cook, nor did many of us eat daily home-cooked meals as we were growing up. The kitchen may still get busy on special occasions – birthdays, anniversaries or religious holidays. However, putting together a family meal often seems like a super-human task requiring several hours of slaving over a dish that gets eaten in minutes and generally tastes only "so-so" compared with the flavor-rich convenience foods we're used to. Thus, many of us feel that cooking is time-consuming, difficult and offers few gastronomic rewards.

This myth still prevents many from preparing their own food at home, although the opposite often holds true: Meals prepared from scratch using fresh, seasonal ingredients and a sprinkling of herbs and spices usually taste more exciting, nourishing and satisfying than processed food. They cost a lot less than take-out or frozen meals and require relatively little energy, skill or equipment to prepare.

As with every new skill we acquire, the beginning is always the hardest, so proceed gradually and go easy on yourself. Start with simple recipes and increase the level of complexity as you gain experience and confidence. Adapt recipes to suit your tastes; substituting ingredients rarely does any damage to the final outcome (except for baking, where one missing egg can make the difference between success or failure).

I am not a professional chef; apart from some *ad hoc* cooking classes I have attended over the years, I was not formally taught to cook. However, my love of good food, coupled with the need to feed a family of five with little time to spare and an eye on costs, drove me to experimentation. With exploration has come this discovery: if you organize yourself just a little, you can eat delicious, healthy meals on a moderate budget and without spending all day in the kitchen!

Meal-planning magic

If you want to cook more meals at home, it helps to plan ahead. This may sound boring, but spending half an hour a week planning what you will eat for the next seven days is a great investment in your health and peace of mind, and can actually save you a lot of time.

Let's face it: many of us start thinking about what we'll eat for dinner an hour or less before we're due to eat. We scramble around in search of ingredients that will make a passable meal; often all we find is an uninspiring collection of limp vegetables or frozen blocks of meat or fish that will take too long to defrost. At this point, many a hungry would-be chef picks up the phone and orders a pizza, followed, perhaps, by ice cream or cookies for dessert. Alas, such meals are tasty, quick and easy but nutritionally poor.

Meal planning can take the fear and loathing out of food preparation and ensure that you eat a varied and healthy diet. Knowing what you will eat and shopping ahead for these meals means that you will not need to ferret around your kitchen cabinets at the last minute. Instead, simply line up the ingredients you bought earlier and proceed to chopping and cooking. The result is a balanced and tasty meal that took less time and nervous energy to prepare than its madly improvised alternative.

Children and partners can also get involved in meal planning by supplying suggestions of favorite healthy dishes. Picky eaters, especially, are more likely to want to help prepare and eat dishes they themselves have asked for.

Lastly, by planning your meals you increase your chances of eating the food you've bought while it's still fresh. Consume the most perishable ingredients first (e.g. lettuce, spinach, mushrooms, ripe avocados), leaving longer-lasting ones (e.g. carrots, onions, beets, green beans) for later in the week. Remember, though, that all vegetables and fruits taste better and contain more nutrients the fresher they are when you eat them.

Once you have decided what to eat, calculate the quantities you will actually need to buy; thus, don't just write "chicken breast" on your shopping list but specify, for instance, "½ pound chicken breast." Shoppers often buy more meat than they need: an adult should eat about four ounces (or 120 grams) of lean meat or fish per meal; people often buy twice as much.

The UK government has launched a campaign called "Love Food, Hate Waste" to help cut back on food waste through meal planning and portion control. The campaign's website (www.lovefoodhatewaste.com) allows shoppers to calculate how much of any food – say, fish, meat or broccoli – they need to buy for a given number of diners. It's often less than you think, so sticking to these guidelines can prevent you over-eating, over-spending and throwing away uneaten leftovers. The website features meal planner and shopping list templates that can be printed out, completed and stuck to the refrigerator for daily guidance. (A similar meal-planning template can be found in Appendix 3 and on this book's website: www.zestforlifediet.com).

To complete your meal planner, start by crossing out the meals that you know you won't eat at home (for instance, weekday lunches if you eat at work). Then cross out any dinners that you might not be having at home (e.g. if you are planning to eat out). Now look at the meals that remain and complete these.

Breakfasts will be fairly predictable, but try to vary them as much as you can. Thus, you might eat a boiled egg with wholegrain toast on Monday, Bircher muesli (p. 238) on Tuesday, Chocolate-hazelnut delight (p. 237) Wednesday, toasted Sourdough bread with Prunella (p. 239) on Thursday, sardines on toast on Friday, Waffles (p. 240) on Saturday and Frittata (pp. 154-155) on Sunday. For each entry, check whether you have all the necessary ingredients (eggs, bread, oats, sardines, etc) and make a note on your shopping list of anything you might need to buy.

Go through the same exercise for lunch and dinner, taking into account the tastes of the people you are catering for, including guests where appropriate. Vary protein sources – fish, beans, meat, eggs, legumes and tofu – and vegetables from one day to the next so that you eat a wide variety of foods. This is the best way of obtaining the broadest possible range of nutrients while avoiding dietary monotony.

When you have eaten your way through seven days' worth of meals, save that week's meal planner in a folder and use it again at a later date. To help you eat seasonally, label your meal-planning sheets by months or seasons (e.g. "Spring/Summer" and "Fall/Winter") and pull them out again at the same time the following year.

The discerning shopper

Without a basic grasp of the way our food affects our health we are too easily tempted by sweet-talking advertisers, alluring packaging and nutritionally ignorant advisers (such as spouses or children!) to buy inappropriate foods. So let's relearn our shopping habits.

Foods that are closest to their natural state and grown nearby are likely to be the most beneficial. You will find these types of foods at a farmers' market or farm store as local farmers only sell seasonal produce. However, even farmers' markets feature imported produce, so if in doubt, check the labels on the crates or ask the person selling it.

Going to a farmers' market regularly and cultivating friendly relationships with stall-holders can be very rewarding. At my local market, for instance, I regularly visit my "organic-vegetable-guy," my "duck-lady" and my "goats' cheese-couple." Not only do I trust these people, having chatted with them and visited their farms; I also know that they value my business and are unlikely to mislead me about the quality of their wares.

This style of shopping does not offer the quick, anonymous retail experience of a supermarket: a visit to a farmers' market can take quite a bit longer as you sniff melons, tap pumpkins and catch up on each other's news. To me, this is an integral part of Mediterranean-style eating.

However, when pressed for time I, too, jog around a grocery store juggling shopping list, left-veering shopping cart and children begging for treats. The experience always leaves me feeling drained and I try to avoid it wherever possible.

Which brings me to supermarkets. They are so convenient: open most hours on most days, selling everything from food to insurance policies, they are a boon for the busy working person with little time to spare, or for someone who only has just enough energy for one-stop shopping. That's fine; I certainly won't tell you not to shop there. But when you do, wear your critical shopper's hat and remember the following tips.

Grocery store survival strategies

- **Do 90% of your shopping along the outer perimeter of the supermarket:** *that is, the aisles selling vegetables, fruits, fish, meat and dairy. If you do venture into the inner aisles where most of the less healthy foods are sold (sugary or alcoholic beverages, cookies, processed oils etc.), make sure you have an exact shopping list of the products you need (e.g. "laundry detergent, matches, garbage bags") and as soon as you have added these to your cart, head quickly back to the safety of the outer perimeter.*

- **Write a detailed shopping list** *before you set off and stick to it; do not let yourself be tempted by special offers for items you do not need. If a "2-for-1" offer happens to correspond with an item on your shopping list, go for it, but first ensure that it is of irreproachable quality.*

- **Never shop on an empty stomach;** *you may yield to unhealthy temptations.*

- **Read labels.** *On fresh produce, check where a fruit or vegetable was grown; if it has travelled half-way around the globe, put it back and find a local alternative. If there is none, it's probably not in season. On packaged foods, check ingredients for industrial fats (e.g. partially hydrogenated vegetable oils), processed sugars (which go by various names, such as sucrose,* *glucose, fructose, high-fructose corn syrup, dextrose, maltodextrin, lactose, etc.) or artificial sweeteners; avoid foods that list them among the top five ingredients – or indeed, foods that list more than five ingredients!*

- **Check expiry dates** *on perishable packaged foods, such as eggs, meat, fish, vegetables and fruits, and always go for the ones that are furthest off. Often these are stacked behind less-fresh foods which the retailer wants to sell first; some careful excavating may be necessary. Be wary of seemingly fresh packaged foods with very distant expiry dates (such as factory-made baked goods); these may contain additives to make them last longer, meaning they might not be as fresh and healthy as they appear.*

- **Be wary of fresh foods that don't perish;** *tomatoes or iceberg lettuce that remain in pristine condition after several weeks in the refrigerator may have been bred for appearance and longevity. They look good, but are they as nutritious as their uglier equivalents that shrivel and wilt after a week? Moreover, do they have any taste?*

- **Taste and smell** *are important considerations: of course we can't go around shops nibbling on foods to test if they're tasty, but we can discreetly use our nose as a flavor indicator. As anyone who has ever bought a perfectly ripe melon, peach, pineapple or vine tomato knows, scent is a key indicator of taste. Fruits and vegetables that don't smell of anything usually don't taste of much either.*

- **Avoid heavily packaged foods;** *generally, the more elaborately packaged a food is, the further removed it is from its natural state. The less packaged, the better – not least for environmental reasons.*

- *As Michael Pollan recommends in his wonderful book,* In Defense of Food: An Eater's Manifesto, **don't buy anything that your great-grandmother would not recognize as food.** *This means: plain yogurt and fresh strawberries rather than strawberry-flavored yogurt-style desserts; plain cocoa and whole milk rather than processed chocolate drinks; oats, raisins and whole nuts instead of processed boxed cereals; and lots of fresh, seasonal vegetables, fruits and legumes. Whenever you're not sure about the healthiness of a food you're about to buy, apply the "great-grandmother-test" and you'll know.*

Seek out seasonal produce

Many of us live in towns and cities and have little awareness of where our fruits and vegetables grow and when they ripen. Imports from around the world ensure that grocery store shelves look much the same in July as they do in December, and so it's

Spring	Summer	Fall	Winter
Fresh, green, tender, eaten raw or cooked	Light, cooling, moist, mostly eaten raw	More warming foods and spices, mostly cooked	Warming foods and spices, usually cooked
asparagus	apricots	apples	avocados
avocados	basil	broccoli	broccoli
basil	beans	brussels sprouts	cabbage (red, kale, savoy, cauliflower, Brussels sprouts, etc)
beans	beets	cabbage (red, cauliflower, Chinese, etc)	
beets	berries	celery (root and stalks)	
berries	broccoli	cranberries	celery (root and stalks)
broccoli	cherries	cucumber	chicory
cabbage (green, white, cauliflower)	cilantro	dates	fennel
	corn	endives	grapefruit
green/spring onions	cucumbers	fennel	greens (spinach, chard)
lettuce	dates	grapes	wild mushrooms
parsley	eggplant	greens (spinach, chard)	mandarins
peas	figs	lettuce	oranges
radish	garlic	mushrooms	onions
rhubarb	grapes	nuts	pears
shallots	melons	mandarins	root vegetables (carrots, parsnips, beets, potatoes)
swiss chard	peas	pears	
spinach	peaches	peppers	
summer squash	peppermint	persimmons	sweet potatoes
	peppers (spicy or sweet)	pomegranates	warming seasonings (e.g. ginger, pepper, mustard)
	plums	quinces	
	summer squash (e.g. zucchini, marrow)	root vegetables (carrots, parsnips, etc)	
	tomatoes	shallots	
	watermelon	sweet potatoes	
		onions	
		warming seasonings (e.g. ginger, pepper, mustard)	
		winter squash	

easy to forget that different crops have different growing seasons and to buy out-of-season produce without realizing it.

If you eat locally grown foods at their peak season you can enjoy a wide diversity of food at its freshest and tastiest. Eating seasonal produce has many benefits besides ripeness and flavor: you avoid paying a premium for food that is scarce and has travelled a long way; you reduce the amount of energy resources and carbon dioxide emissions needed to grow and transport food; you support the local economy; and you reconnect with nature's cycles, experiencing consciously the ebb and flow of the seasons.

The best way of ensuring that your produce is seasonal is to buy it from local producers. If you shop in a supermarket, read the labels that tell you where the produce was grown. If it's from your country or a neighboring one, then it's probably in season; if it has flown half-way around the globe, it is not. An exception to the seasonal-foods-rule are those that do not grow at all in your part of the world, for example, chocolate, green tea or citrus fruit. The table opposite is intended to serve as a guide to seasonal food choices.

The anti-cancer pantry

I admit it: I'm a hoarder. My family often jokes that if we were snowed-in we could live off my provisions for at least four weeks – which is probably true, albeit an unlikely weather scenario where I live. My excuse for having substantial food stocks is that I live in the countryside and don't want to drive four miles to the nearest shop just because I need a jar of beans. Moreover, having a wide array of long-lasting foods to choose from helps me keep meals varied.

Keeping a well-stocked pantry makes it easier to create quick, nutritious meals at home. Even if you aren't a meal planner, having healthy food choices in your kitchen, pantry and freezer makes it easier to prepare healthy meals quickly.

In the shopping list template in Appendix 4, which you can also download from this book's website (www.zestforlifediet.com) I suggest a list of anti-cancer pantry items to get you started. Make copies of this list and display a blank one at a visible place in your kitchen so you can mark items you need to buy. You can also make a note of any foods you need to get for the week's meals generated on your meal planner.

Eating on the move

No matter how disciplined we are at home, our good intentions can fly out the window when we are out and about. Rather than risk the guilty funk that ensues when we break new-found virtuous habits, you can prepare for these situations.

First of all: if you do make a transgression – for instance, eating a donut because you were hungry and sitting in a meeting where nothing else was available – don't beat yourself up. Negative or punishing thoughts will only make you feel worse.

Transgressions happen, and as long they are occasional only, they won't make that much difference to your overall wellbeing. Indeed, if they're unavoidable, you might as well enjoy them for the very rare treats they have become!

You can counteract glitches by compensating with healthy foods: thus, an ill-advised donut in the morning can be offset by one or two fresh apricots, an apple, a tub of plain yogurt with chopped fruit or nuts and raisins as an afternoon snack.

Healthy travel snacks

If you are going to be away from home for more than a day, why not carry a "travel pack" of healthy snacks that includes the following:

- Resealable plastic bags filled with **dried fruit and nuts** (make your own trail mix – commercial nuts often taste stale)
- **Chopped fruit** and a wooden toothpick for easy snacking (melon cubes, grapes, oranges, pineapple, kiwi, etc) in a tightly sealable tub
- **Chopped vegetables** (carrot sticks, pepper strips, cucumber slices, broccoli or cauliflower florets), possibly with a tub of hummus, sardine salad or herby cottage cheese for dipping
- **Whole fresh fruit** that can be eaten easily without requiring preparation (apples, tangerines, bananas, fresh apricots, peaches)
- **Home-made wholegrain sandwiches** containing vegetables (e.g. tomatoes, lettuce, cucumber) and a good source of protein (fresh goats' cheese, cut-up falafels, salmon, sardines, tuna mousse, cold chicken breast or other left-over lean meat)
- **Dark chocolate** as a special treat

If you plan to stay somewhere else for more than two nights – for instance, on vacation in a hotel, a self-catering apartment or with friends or relatives – it may be useful to bring some of your favorite foods to maintain your healthy eating habits. If you do not, you may find that your digestion grinds to a halt, your energy levels drop and you feel generally unwell. If you tell your hosts that you have special dietary needs, most people won't mind; if anything, they'll be impressed that you are taking responsibility for your health, and relieved that they don't have to.

My travelling vacation store cupboard usually includes:

- nut milk (at least one or two packs to last me until I can buy more locally)
- oat or rye crackers to avoid having to eat the white bread typically served in hotels
- herbal and green tea bags
- a few cans of sardines
- nut butter (hazelnut, almond or cashew)

Don't stress out when you eat out

Eating in a restaurant – whether for business or pleasure – can be an occasion for relaxed enjoyment or nutritional anxiety; it all depends on where you go and what you order.

Eateries promising a fast or inexpensive dining experience – especially when they are part of a big chain – are best regarded with skepticism. Whether they serve pizza, pasta, burgers or ethnic cuisine, fast food is usually prepared in advance or in a rush and nutritional value may get sacrificed in the name of speed and efficiency.

However, you don't need to go to three-star restaurants to get good food; most establishments that don't belong to a chain and do "from scratch" cooking offer good nutrition at reasonable prices. Many family-run ethnic neighborhood restaurants – such as Lebanese, French, Italian, Greek, Indian, Asian or Mexican – use fresh ingredients. Here, your best bets are vegetable-rich *hors d'oeuvres* such as soups, salads or roasted vegetables, and main dishes that include fish or lean meat, legumes and, again, plenty of vegetables. You can ask the chef to substitute French fries, pasta or white rice with a green vegetable or salad. Most restaurants also provide side servings of salad or vegetables at moderate cost.

Skip the bread basket – a cruel temptation as you sit hungrily waiting to be served. The bread served in restaurants is generally made with white flour and rarely offers a memorable gourmet experience, so just say "no." I often hand the bread back to the waiter explaining that I don't want to be tempted; I usually get an understanding smile.

When it comes to dessert, I'm a bit more relaxed. If you choose something healthy, like pears poached in red wine, that's great, but occasional indulgences are fine, too. If you want to have a more decadent dessert, why not share it with your dining partner? And make sure to savor every spoonful of this rare treat.

Time saving tips

Many people do not cook meals from scratch because they haven't got the time. Or so they think!

In fact, preparing a meal using fresh ingredients need not take longer than using processed food, especially if you plan ahead and avoid last-minute scrambling for ingredients. A study[1] of Californian families preparing weeknight dinners showed that convenience foods did not significantly speed up meal preparation time: home-cooked meals made mostly with fresh ingredients took just as long to prepare – 52 minutes on average – as meals consisting largely of commercial convenience foods. Heavy use of commercial foods saved, on average 10-12 minutes of the time spent washing, chopping and stirring, but did not reduce total preparation time.

Meal-preparation time savers

- **Meal planning** *(see p. 98). Plan meals ahead of time and shop for them; this will limit time spent shopping to one big weekly shopping trip and one or two stops at specialist shops for highly perishable foods such as fish, eggs or meat.*

- **Strategic shopping:** *Get to know the lay-out of the shops you most regularly frequent so you can buy what you need and leave as quickly as you can. Nothing is more frustrating and time-consuming than traipsing up and down unknown aisles in search of an elusive product.*

- **Bulk cooking:** *When you prepare a meal, make two or three times more than you plan to eat and freeze the rest. Later, this can be defrosted at a moment's notice: your very own home-made convenience food! All it requires is large pots, some storage containers and a freezer.*

- **Use a crock pot (slow cooker):** *These counter-top appliances are a godsend for time-starved cooks. Simply place all necessary ingredients in the pot, work or run errands and return as many as six hours later to a delicious ready-to-eat dish that requires little more intervention than some light seasoning. Additional advantages of crock pots are that they cook food at low temperatures (generally at a range of 175°F/80°C to 195°F/90°C), reducing the risk of carcinogenic by-products and using less electricity than most conventional heat sources. Furthermore, cooking the meal in a single pot reduces washing up, and the low cooking temperature and glazed pot make cleaning very easy. From a gastronomic perspective, nothing beats the comfort provided by a dish whose flavors have infused over several hours.*

- **Ready-to-use fresh produce:** *Most supermarkets sell chopped fresh vegetables, salad greens and fruit. So if you haven't got the time to peel, pluck, wash and dry produce, vegetables* *or lettuce from a bag — ideally the one with the remotest "best-before" date — are vastly preferable to tinned vegetables or no vegetables at all!*

- **Salad dressings and sauces:** *Make batches of salad dressing (p. 234), Basic tomato sauce (p. 226) or Turmeric chutney (p. 230) and keep these on stand-by in refrigerator and freezer. This way, even if you haven't had time to plan your meal you can rustle up a quick and tasty vegetable, salad or pasta dish without missing out on nutrients.*

- **Organize your kitchen:** *It should only contain the tools you use frequently, and they should always be stored in the same place. Hunting high and low for that elusive apple corer can waste precious time.*

- **Get help:** *Any able-bodied person from the age of six upwards should be able to perform at least menial kitchen jobs which will speed up meal preparation. Enlist help from family members for basic peeling, chopping and stirring, washing up during meal preparation or, at the very least, to set the table.*

- **Avoid distractions:** *Turn off the TV and don't answer the phone while cooking; this will allow you to give your whole attention to the meal preparation at hand, and won't get in the way of talking amiably with your kitchen helper.*

- **Tried and tested favorites:** *When you're in a hurry to make a meal, don't experiment with new ingredients or recipes. Stick to the ones you know.*

The family meal: An unexpected time-saver

Imagine a family where Mom eats a low-fat diet, Dad wants red meat, the 13-year-old daughter is a vegetarian and the 9-year old son hates vegetables. In this increasingly common scenario, each person insists on their own dish. Moreover, in many families, the children eat different foods, and at different times, than the adults.

Meals at which everyone shares the same dish – as humans have done since the dawn of civilization – reduce the time spent preparing separate dishes and increase overall conviviality. Few things are more conducive to strengthening social and familial bonds than sharing a meal – the *same* meal. It's the Mediterranean way.

In addition to being enjoyable, there is increasing scientific evidence that family meals boost their participants' physical and psychological well-being. Thus, children who regularly eat with their family consume more vegetables and fruits and are less likely to be overweight, smoke or take drugs, or develop eating disorders. Even children with chronic asthma do better when they regularly eat relaxed, interactive family meals! [1a]

Accommodating everybody's wishes will require some negotiating and advance planning; considerations such as "health" and "budget" should outweigh purely flavor-driven preferences and meals should alternate so there's something for everyone.

Cost savings

Many people think that eating a healthy diet is a luxury and that convenience foods are cheaper than meals cooked from scratch. Granted, rising prices have increased households' food costs, but eating healthily doesn't have to be expensive. If anything, cooking your own meals will help you keep costs low.

This is particularly true of the Mediterranean diet which relies on relatively inexpensive vegetables, fruits, legumes, nuts, seeds, whole grains and eggs, and largely avoids more expensive items such as meat and sugary or processed foods. Indeed, a Canadian study found that women eating a Mediterranean diet did not have higher food costs than those eating a typical North American diet[2]. While they spent more on vegetables, fruits, legumes, nuts, seeds, oil, fish and poultry, they spent less on red meat, refined grain products, desserts, candy and fast food.

It's also time to debunk the popular myth that pre-prepared meals cost less than home-made meals. A British consumer advocacy group compared the cost of processed foods with their home-made equivalents[3]. They found that, compared to the home-made version, shop-bought shepherd's pie was 61% more expensive, commercial rice pudding was 55% dearer, ready-made lasagna cost 48% more and pre-packaged fruit crumble was 34% more expensive.

Some dishes – such as chicken nuggets or fishcakes – were cheaper to buy ready-made than to prepare at home, which makes you wonder what actually goes into these to make them so inexpensive!

Healthy eating on a budget

- **Meal planning (yes, again!):** *Plan your meals around your budget, make a shopping list and stick to it; do not make impulse purchases based on alluring advertisements or sudden cravings.*

- **Keep convenience meals to a minimum:** *These are expensive and nutritionally poor. Stock some inexpensive staples such as legumes, wholegrain pasta and tomatoes in jars so you can rustle up quick, healthy meals at a moment's notice.*

- **Shop around:** *Compare prices to find out which shops offer the best deals. Fruit and vegetables are often cheaper at farmers' markets than in supermarkets. When buying staples such as beans or olive oil, go for less-known brands, which are unlikely to differ vastly in quality from the more expensive names. Don't fall for "2-for-1" offers unless they are on your shopping list.*

- **Buy in bulk:** *In some cases — especially at health-food shops — it is more cost-effective to buy dry goods loose from self-service bins rather than purchasing sealed packages. At farmers' markets, buying a whole tray of peaches or zucchini is often less expensive than buying them individually weighed. Large bags of frozen vegetables and fruits often cost less than smaller portions, and since they are frozen, you can use as much as you need and return the rest to the freezer for later. Bulk shopping and bulk cooking go hand-in-hand; when you see a good bulk price for something, buy it, cook it and freeze it; you'll feel so smart!*

- **Do your research:** *More and more consumer advocacy services offer advice on food in magazines or on the internet. You may discover unknown brands sold at cheaper prices that are of superior quality than well-known, more expensive products.*

- **DIY:** *Instead of buying pre-chopped vegetables or fruits, get them whole, wash and chop them yourself and pack them into containers or resealable plastic bags for refrigerator or freezer. Make popsicles from frozen fruit juice or pureed fruit; these are usually tastier and healthier than their shop-bought counterparts, at a fraction of the cost.*

- **Shop for seasonal, locally grown fresh fruit and vegetables.** *Fruits and vegetables that are not in season where we live are often transported over long distances and so can be rather expensive. Local, seasonal produce is cheaper and also better for our environment. Don't let advertisers fool you into buying exotic and costly "super-foods." It is important to eat a wide variety of fruits and vegetables; no single fruit or vegetable is superior to the rest.*

A handful of tools

Cooking is often described as an "art" or a "science," and this can intimidate beginners. Rest assured, to prepare the recipes in this book you need to be neither a scientist, nor an artist. All you need are a selection of fresh ingredients, some basic tools and an openness to explore new ways of preparing and eating food. Each recipe in this book has been designed for people with limited culinary experience, time, and cooking equipment. Having said this, it's easier to cook quick, tasty meals if you own the following utensils.

Basic kitchen equipment

- **Three to four good-quality kitchen knives** *of different sizes (e.g., a small paring knife, a small knife with a serrated edge to cut tomatoes or eggplants; a large knife with a slightly curved blade for chopping herbs, vegetables, onions, etc; and another straight-bladed, long one for cutting large objects such as watermelons). Sharpen these regularly; not only do they work better; you are also less likely to cut yourself with a sharp knife than with a blunt one.*

- **A "microplane" grater** *for grating lemon or orange zest (use untreated fruits only), ginger, garlic, chocolate, nutmeg and anything else that needs to be finely grated. Its small, flat teeth result in more evenly and finely grated foods than traditional box graters and also entail less wastage. Available from good kitchen suppliers.*

- **Two large chopping boards:** *Bamboo boards are more resistant than wooden ones and can even go in the dishwasher, making them more convenient and hygienic to use.*

- **A blender or liquidizer:** *A hand-held pureeing device will suffice for most jobs, but an upright blender with a strong motor and a large jug with a volume of about three pints (1.5 liters) is best. Use to make soups, sauces, purees, fruit coulis, shakes and smoothies.*

- **A basic food processor:** *You don't need a super-deluxe food processor with 101 attachments. Indeed, mine only has three: an S-shaped blade for chopping and grinding, a disk with a slicing insert and another with a grating insert. It has a tiny motor and stores easily in a deep kitchen drawer.*

- **An electric whisk** *for mixing pancake batter, cake or bread dough, for beating egg whites or making mayonnaise. A basic model is sufficient for most uses.*

- **A single- or double-bladed half-moon shaped herb chopper with wooden handles ("mezzaluna")** *for chopping fresh herbs, especially when you need to chop large amounts for dishes like* tabouleh. *Can also be used to chop nuts, chocolate, onions or garlic.*

- **The usual:** *Can opener, garlic press, potato peeler, apple corer, balloon whisk, rubber or silicone spatula to scrape residues out of mixing bowls. You may have some of these already, lurking at the back of your drawers. If not, they can be found in any hardware store or supermarket.*

Of pots and pans

There is widespread concern over the potential cancer risks of non-stick cookware. Traditional non-stick coatings are made with chemicals thought to be carcinogenic, such as PTFE (polytetrafluoro ethylene) and PFOA (perfluorooctanoic acid), and that may be released when non-stick cookware is overheated. Health authorities advise against heating non-stick cookware above 480°F (250°C), especially when empty; moreover, it should not be used for high-temperature broiling or cooking.

Traditional cast-iron pans contain no synthetic materials, are extremely hard wearing and conduct heat evenly. Once these pans are well-seasoned, food rarely sticks to them (unless the pan is too hot). They are also very easy to clean – soak briefly in water and wash with a sponge or soft brush. Avoid using soap or detergent, as these will remove the seasoning from cast-iron cookware. Their only drawback is that they can be quite heavy and you may need to use both hands – and a thick oven mitt – to lift them.

Stainless steel pans are not particularly suitable for frying as food sticks to them easily. For cooking pots, however, stainless steel and enamel are my favorite materials; they are safe, flavor-neutral, hard-wearing and easy to clean.

Water-boiling is best done in traditional stainless steel or enamel stove-top kettles, or even just a casserole with a lid. If you prefer using an electric kettle, avoid plastic kettles and use a stainless steel one instead.

Seasoning secrets

Picture this scene: you're in the kitchen, cooking, say, a lentil stew. The recipe says: "season to taste." You add some salt. Hmmm – it still doesn't taste right. So you give it a grind of pepper. Something's still missing.

If at this point you're tempted to add more salt, think again. You've already added "S" and "A" – what you may need is another "S," an "F" and a "U" to make that casserole taste just right. Lest you wonder, I'm talking about "F.A.S.S.U." – the magic acronym for seasoning your food! (It stands for **F**at, **A**cidity, **S**weetness, **S**altiness and **U**mami. We'll come back to them shortly.)

Taste is personal, and people's ideas of what tastes good vary widely. Highly individual factors affect how you like a dish to taste: If you have a cold, are going through chemotherapy or if you were brought up to enjoy strong or very flavors, your idea of "tasty" will be heavily influenced by these factors. So "seasoning to taste" is about what *you* think tastes good.

It is not only our own sense of taste that can change; the flavor of a dish also evolves while it is cooking and so it's useful to *keep tasting* as you're cooking. Some flavors – for instance, spices – grow stronger the longer they are cooked; others –

fresh herbs, for example – lose some of their aroma through lengthy cooking and are best added at the end.

Many of us are so used to processed food (which often contains synthetic flavor enhancers) that we think anything we cook ourselves tastes boring by comparison. Moreover, people who are new to cooking and seasoning may not always trust their taste buds; they may sense that "something is missing" but can't put their finger on what it is.

In her cancer-recovery cookbook *One Bite at a Time*, health-food chef and writer Rebecca Katz describes the magical workings of "F.A.S.S." I have added a fifth letter, "U," which stands for *umami*, a concept we explore below. To have a fully-rounded flavor, most dishes need to contain a little of each of the following elements:

FASSU

- **Fat** *is needed to give food a satisfying mouth-feel and to convey and develop the flavors of the dish; this is why fat-free or low-fat food often tastes bland and unsatisfying.*

- **Acidity** *brings a dish to life. Have you noticed how just a few drops of lemon juice in a soup seem to wake up the whole dish? Other sources of acidity are tomatoes, acidic fruits like orange or kiwi and liquid seasonings such as balsamic, red-wine or apple-cider vinegar, or white wine.*

- *As for* **sweetness**, *while savory dishes should not taste sugary, a touch of honey or the addition of fruit can bring a mellow, rounded flavor to a savory stew or salad. I often add a hint of acacia honey to salad dressings, tomato-based sauces and marinades to open them up. Sweetness is not only derived from sugar, but also comes from slowly-stewed vegetables such as onions, carrots, beets, bell peppers and even broccoli. The more you chew vegetables and legumes (aim for 30 times per mouthful) the more these foods' sweet flavor comes to the fore.*

- **Salt:** *You may be surprised that I advocate the use of salt. True, eaten in excess (e.g., when we eat a lot of processed food) salt can increase the risk of stomach cancer and raise blood pressure. (The American Institute for Cancer Research/World Cancer Research Fund (AICR/WCRF) recommends we consume no more than 6 grams of salt, or 2.4 grams sodium, a day.) However, for healthy people eating a diet of unprocessed whole foods and drinking sufficient liquids, a small amount of salt added during cooking poses little threat. You can further use onions, garlic, herbs (e.g. oregano, dill, thyme, rosemary, peppermint, parsley) and spices (e.g. cinnamon, coriander, turmeric) to boost a dish's flavor.*

- **Umami:** *If you want to reduce salt but don't want to lose the oomph it offers you're probably looking for* umami *(the Japanese word for "flavor" or "taste").* Umami *adds a meaty flavor to a meal thanks to the presence of glutamic acid, a naturally occurring amino acid in meats, cheese, broth, and other protein-heavy foods. There are several ways to boost the* umami *taste in a meal. One is to add ingredients rich in glutamic acid, such as Italian hard cheeses Parmesan or pecorino; red wine; tomato juice, paste or ketchup; and tamari or fish-based sauces like Worcestershire and Thai fish sauce. Another is to use foods rich in compounds that contribute to the* umami *taste, such as seafood, dried or preserved fish (such as anchovies) and meat, and broths made from bones.*

  Vegetarians can obtain umami *flavor by adding mushrooms (especially when dried) and dried sea vegetables to their food. Try adding dried kelp, dulse or nori flakes (from health food shops or Asian supermarkets) to your food instead of salt, and flavor soups or stews with arame, kombu and wakame seaweeds. These not only taste delicious, they also contain thyroid-supporting iodine, a vast array of essential minerals, anti-inflammatory compounds and lignans.*

And now, let's cook! *Bon appétit!*

Summary: 10 Principles Of Dietary Cancer Prevention

1. Eat 5–10 portions of fresh vegetables and fruits daily and regularly eat legumes, nuts and seeds. At least two-thirds of the food on your plate should be of plant origin.

2. Eat foods that calm inflammation: Most vegetables, fruits, herbs, spices and foods rich in omega-3 fatty acids (oily fish, walnuts, flax seed, leafy greens, omega-3-enriched eggs). **Avoid foods that increase inflammation:** Sugar, refined grain products, hydrogenated fats, oils rich in omega-6 fatty acids (corn, sunflower, safflower oil).

3. Variety is the spice of life. Eat a wide diversity of fresh, natural foods, varying your choices daily. Eating a wide variety of healthy foods offers greater nutritional benefits than eating just a handful, no matter how healthy these may be. Varying your foods along with the changing seasons will help you to obtain the widest-possible variety of nutrients.

4. Blood-sugar balance: Minimize your intake of sugar, sweetened foods/drinks and refined grains (e.g. white flour, pasta and rice) or foods made with these (e.g. cookies, cakes, rice crackers). Replace high-glycemic carbohydrates with low-glycemic alternatives (see pp. 39-43). Retrain your taste buds to accept less-sweet tastes, and when you do use sweetener, sparingly use acacia honey, date sugar or molasses.

5. Eat healthy protein at every meal; protein helps to curb snacking, balance blood sugar and maintain muscle mass during illness. Meat is not the only source of protein; fish, eggs, legumes, soy foods, nuts, seeds and many vegetables also provide protein.

6. Avoid industrially manufactured foods that are heavily processed, contain man-made flavorings, colorings, sweeteners, preservatives and fillers, are elaborately packaged and have remote expiry dates.

7. Avoid unhealthy chemicals. High-temperature barbecuing, grilling or frying of meat increases the risk of some cancers; cook meat gently and avoid preserved meats. Avoid moldy foods and limit peanuts. Avoid canned food and drinks and don't microwave food in plastic containers. Chose organic foods where indicated (p. 48).

8. Prepare most meals from scratch using unprocessed ingredients. This takes a little more time than buying packaged food but provides more nutrients, cost savings and, for many, a deep sense of satisfaction.

9. Eat regular meals and chew your food thoroughly to ensure optimal digestion, nutrient absorption and mealtime satisfaction. Take time to relax and enjoy your meals.

10. Drink water: It hydrates and cleanses our bodies without adding calories or chemicals. Fresh vegetable and fruit juices are fine occasionally, but whole fruits or vegetables are preferable. Green and white tea may have cancer-protective properties, so drink these if you enjoy their taste.

Zest for Life
Mediterranean
Anti-Cancer Recipes

Snacks and hors d'oeuvres

Traditional Mediterranean cuisine is an informal style of cooking and eating. Formally structured three-course meals may feature on restaurant menus, but in most casual eateries or homes people eat light meals consisting of a main dish accompanied perhaps by a side vegetable or salad and rounded off with a light dessert or sweet nibble.

In many Mediterranean countries small, informal dishes are eaten with drinks, as an *hors d'oeuvre*, or even a main meal. In Spain these are called *tapas*, in Turkey, Greece and Lebanon they are known as *meze* and in Italy they are referred to as *antipasti*.

These usually consist of savory dishes involving vegetables (e.g. tomatoes, artichoke hearts, onions, garlic, eggplant, mushrooms), cheese and olives, garbanzos and almonds, meat, fish and seafood, and are eaten with toothpicks or on small slices of bread.

Since I like this informal style of eating I have dispensed with *hors d'oeuvres* in this book. However, in the section that follows I suggest a variety of small, savory dishes inspired by these Mediterranean tidbits.

These, as well as soups and salads, in the following two sections, can easily be served as *hors d'oeuvres* if you are planning a more formal meal.

Artichoke-heart *petits fours*

2.2lb/1kg artichoke hearts
(fleshy base only, without
leaves), frozen, or from a
jar or a BPA-free tin

7fl oz/1 scant cup/200ml
Basic tomato sauce (p.
226)

20 black olives, pitted and
cut in halves

10 oil-packed anchovy
fillets, rinsed

2oz/50g pine nuts

2oz/50g grated ewes' milk
cheese

basil leaves to garnish

These savory nibbles are inspired by tiny sweet French cakes called *petits fours*. Artichoke hearts provide useful support for almost any topping: tapenade, sun-dried tomatoes and feta cheese; Roquefort and walnuts; mushrooms and spinach; figs and Parma ham – the list goes on. Anything that tastes good on a pizza tastes good on artichoke hearts. I've gone for a very Mediterranean mix of flavors: tomatoes, olives, mushrooms, basil, pine nuts and melted cheese. Serve, *petits fours*-style, on a pretty serving platter with drinks, or as an *hors d'oeuvre* accompanied by lightly tossed arugula or other salad greens, counting two per person. Makes about 10-12 petits-fours.

If using frozen artichoke hearts, bring water to the boil in a large pot. Once boiling, add salt and artichoke hearts. Cook until soft, 8-10 minutes. If using artichoke hearts from a jar, simply drain, rinse and pat dry; no need to cook these.

Place empty artichoke hearts on a baking tray, if necessary slicing away thin wedges underneath to stabilize them. Fill with tomato sauce, olives, anchovies, pine nuts or anything else you might wish to add. Sprinkle lightly with cheese and place under a medium-hot grill for 10 minutes.

Once the cheese is melted and golden and the filling warmed through, remove from oven, transfer to serving platter or individual plates and serve immediately.

Savory aperitif loaf

This type of savory loaf – often served in France with pre-dinner drinks – is moist, nourishing and an excellent vehicle for sunny Mediterranean flavors. Olive oil replaces butter, cheese and eggs provide protein, and herbs and vegetables add taste and protective plant chemicals. This loaf is quick to prepare and easy to transport, making it an ideal addition to any lunchbox or picnic. It also makes a great in-between snack or a satisfying accompaniment to a simple soup. Using muffin molds halves baking time. Makes 1 loaf or 10-12 muffins.

Preheat oven to 350°F (180°C) and oil a rectangular loaf tin. In a bowl, mix flour and baking powder and make a hollow at the center. Add eggs, olive oil and milk and whisk into a smooth batter. Add chopped olives, tomatoes, cheese, oregano, turmeric, pepper and garlic and combine gently with a fork, being careful not to break up the cheese.

Pour batter into the loaf tin, scatter with pine nuts and dust with paprika powder. Place in preheated oven; bake loaf for 45-50 minutes (muffins for 20-25 minutes), or until a skewer or toothpick inserted into the center comes out clean.

Cool for 5 minutes, then turn out onto a wire rack and cool at least 30 minutes more.

Variations

- Mozzarella (instead of feta), sundried tomatoes, pine nuts and basil (replacing oregano) yield a more Italian aroma.
- Vegetables such as bell peppers, mushrooms, zucchini or asparagus can also be added (they should be finely chopped and cooked for 5-10 minutes in a skillet with a little olive oil to reduce their moisture content).

5½ oz/heaped 1 cup/150g wholegrain spelt or wheat flour

2 tsp baking powder

3 eggs

3.5fl oz/scant ½ cup/100ml olive oil

5fl oz/scant cup/150ml unsweetened almond milk

1¾ oz/½ cup/50g black olives, chopped

1 ¾ oz/½ cup/50g sundried tomatoes, chopped

5 ¼oz/150g feta or other ewes' milk cheese, cubed

1 tsp oregano (fresh or dried)

1 tsp turmeric

1 clove garlic, crushed

2 tbsp pine nuts

dusting of paprika powder

freshly ground black pepper

Roast peppers with garlic and olives

4 red, yellow or green bell peppers (or a mix of all three)

6-8 cloves garlic, skins left on

16 black olives, coarsely chopped

1 teaspoon capers, rinsed

squeeze of lemon juice

4 tbsp best-quality olive oil

salt & freshly ground pepper

This delicious Provençal side dish can be enjoyed on its own, as an *hors d'oeuvre* or as an accompaniment to grilled fish, meat or eggs. You can double the quantity and keep some on stand-by; in the refrigerator and well-coated with olive oil, these keep for at least a week, getting increasingly delicious as the flavors infuse. Serves 4.

Preheat grill on high setting. Place whole peppers and garlic cloves in their skins on a baking sheet and slide under hot grill.

Roast until the peppers' skin starts to discolor (about 5 minutes). Then, with a pair of kitchen tongs, rotate them slightly to expose a fresh patch of skin to the heat. Continue like this for about 15-20 minutes until the peppers' skin is evenly darkened. Turn over the garlic cloves once during this time.

Meanwhile, chop olives and drain and rinse capers. Remove peppers from oven, tip them into a container with a tight-fitting lid and close. (The steam coming off the hot peppers will soften the skins and make them easier to remove.) After 10 minutes, open container, peel the burnt skins off the peppers and remove seeds. Cut peppers into broad strips and place in serving dish.

Squeeze garlic cloves out of their skins and add to the peeled peppers. Drizzle with olive oil and lemon juice and season with salt and pepper. Garnish with sliced olives and capers and marinate in the refrigerator for at least 1 hour before serving.

This is delicious sprinkled with chopped summer herbs – such as basil or oregano – and lightly toasted pine nuts.

Marinated feta cheese

More of a condiment than a dish, this fragrant marinated cheese comes in handy in many unexpected ways. Sprinkle it over salads, vegetables and soups (e.g. Greek bean stew, p. 191), pile it onto pizzas (e.g. Eggplant "pizzas," p. 216) frittatas or tarts, spoon it into a crisp slice of sourdough toast or simply enjoy it on its own with pre-dinner drinks. If you want this to keep longer, use dried herbs (oregano, *herbes de Provence*), but if you plan to have it within 24 hours, fresh herbs provide a vibrant aroma that dried herbs just can't match.

Remove cheese from its package and drain off brine; pat dry with a paper towel. Cube to the desired size and place in serving bowl.

In a mixing bowl, combine olive oil, lemon zest and juice, garlic, herbs and pepper and whisk with a fork until smooth. Pour this over cubed cheese and mix gently, being careful not to break up the crumbly cheese. Leave to marinate for at least one hour to allow flavors to develop. Keeps 2-3 days in a tightly sealed container.

7oz/200g plain ewes' milk feta cheese

4 tbsp best-quality olive oil

zest and juice of ½ lemon

1 clove garlic, crushed

freshly chopped herbs (oregano, mint or parsley or a mix of all three); dried herbs are fine if fresh herbs aren't available

freshly ground black pepper

Tapenade and Sardinade

*7oz/heaped 1 cup/200g
pitted black olives, rinsed*

*2 tbsp capers, rinsed
thoroughly of their brine*

*2 olive-oil-packed anchovy
fillets, rinsed*

½ tsp thyme or savory

1 clove garlic, crushed

2 tbsp olive oil

1 tbsp lemon juice

*freshly ground black
pepper*

*7oz/200g whole sardines
in olive oil from a jar or
BPA-free tin, drained*

½ onion, finely chopped

1 rib celery, finely chopped

1 tsp capers

1 tbsp Dijon mustard

*salt & freshly ground black
pepper to taste*

*large pinch herbes de
Provence*

lemon juice

*freshly ground black
pepper*

chopped chives

These two gutsy Provençal pastes are very simple to make and wonderfully versatile.

Tapenade

Delicious as a dip with raw vegetables, a sandwich base for sardines or fresh goats' cheese, slathered onto steamed, bland vegetables (carrots, squash or turnips), spooned onto an omelet or mashed with the yolks of hard-boiled eggs for devilled eggs. Use green olives for a milder taste.

Place olives, capers, anchovies, herbs and crushed garlic in a food processor and process until smooth. With the food processor running, pour in the olive oil in a steady stream to form a smooth paste. Mix in the lemon juice and season to taste with pepper. Stored in a tightly sealed jar in the refrigerator, this will keep for at least 2 weeks.

Sardinade

This is delicious on toast, in avocado halves, atop a mixed salad or piled, canapé-style, onto cucumber slices as an aperitif nibble.

Combine all the ingredients, except lemon juice and pepper, in a small bowl and mash with a fork. If you whizz this in a blender it will yield a smoother texture. Season to taste with pepper and lemon juice. Sprinkle with finely chopped chives.

Marinated mushrooms

A delicious snack with an aperitif, these mushrooms can also be enjoyed as topping for "Pizza" (p. 200), Artichoke heart *petits fours* (p. 118), or tossed into a salad.

Wipe earth or grit off the mushrooms with a damp cloth; do not wash them as this will make them soggy. Cut off the stalks. Leave the mushrooms whole unless they are very large, in which case you can halve or quarter them.

In a skillet on medium heat, warm 1 tablespoon olive oil and gently cook mushrooms and shallots for 5 minutes until the mushrooms are soft but still *al dente*.

While the mushrooms are cooking, whisk the remaining ingredients – olive oil, vinegar, garlic, salt, pepper, parsley and *herbes de Provence* – in a medium mixing bowl. As soon as the mushrooms are soft, tip them into the dressing and toss well. Cool and refrigerate for at least 4-5 hours, preferably overnight. These keep for up to a week in a tightly sealed container.

If serving as pre-dinner nibbles, serve in a bowl, a few mushrooms speared with toothpicks.

1.1lb/500g chestnut or button mushrooms

7 tbsp olive oil

1 shallot, finely chopped

3 tbsp red wine vinegar

1 clove garlic, crushed

2 tbsp chopped parsley

pinch of herbes de Provence

salt, pepper

Salads

If you can obtain high-quality, fresh vegetables, salads are the very essence of Life Energy. At any time of year – even winter! – a mixed salad can offer seemingly endless sensations: crisp greens, buttery avocados, tangy apples, crunchy nuts, sweet berries, earthy beets, pungent onions and garlic, spicy herbs, peppery olive oil and sharp lemon juice being just a few.

Salads are also a great opportunity to pack in extra nutrients: why stop at lettuce and tomatoes when you can throw in dried cranberries, feta cheese, walnuts and broccoli sprouts? Or toasted sunflower seeds, a few leftover sundried tomatoes, olives and a few crumbs of feta cheese? I sometimes have a bit of quiet fun trying to see just how many healthy, tasty ingredients I can sneak into a salad before my family starts to complain. So far, they haven't noticed.

Try to stick with seasonal salad ingredients: in winter, choose grated cabbage of all colors, cress, winter greens (e.g. arugula, *frisée* lettuce, endives, bitter red lettuce), grated root vegetables (carrots, raw or cooked beets, celeriac), winter fruit (apples, pears, oranges), cooked legumes (lentils, beans, garbanzos) and nuts.

In summer, choose from nature's bounty: tomatoes, bell peppers, summer lettuce, sweet raw peas, green beans, spring onions, asparagus, zucchini, cherries, grapes, melon balls – don't be shy.

Dressings are another place to let your imagination run wild: by varying oils (olive, walnut, and hazelnut are my favorites), acids (lemon juice, balsamic, sherry or red-wine vinegar) and herbs and spices (basil, tarragon, cilantro, mint, parsley, garlic, ginger, turmeric) you can make every salad taste unique. (See salad dressings on p. 234).

Why not make larger batches of salad dressings and store these in the refrigerator? This way, you can rustle up a salad in no time and won't have to worry about mixing a dressing.

Bean and sardine salad

This recipe is inspired by the classic Tuscan bean-and-tuna salad, *tonno e fagioli*. I use omega-3-rich sardines instead of tuna because of the pollutants large fish can contain. This is delicious on its own as an appetizer, but equally good lightly mashed and wrapped – cigar-style – in romaine lettuce leaves or piled on wholegrain toast as a healthy snack.

Tuscans would use cannellini beans for this recipe but I like a mix of legumes – garbanzos, navy, red kidney or black-eyed beans – which tastes just as good and looks more interesting. If cooking the beans from scratch, add some sage to the cooking water for flavor and ease of digestion. If you're pressed for time, beans from a jar are fine, although they'll taste slightly less fresh and fall apart more easily when you are tossing the salad. Serves 4-6.

If using dried beans, start a day earlier and follow instructions on p. 186. If using pre-cooked beans from a jar or tin, drain these in a sieve and rinse thoroughly under cold tap water.

Open sardine tin or jar and drain oil. Tip sardines into a small bowl and flake lightly with a fork. Prepare Italian dressing (p. 234).

In a large bowl, combine chopped onion, garlic, celery, pepper, parsley, lemon zest and olives or capers. Add drained beans and sardines. Now pour the dressing over and lightly toss until all ingredients are coated, but taking care not to mash or crush the beans and the fish. Refrigerate for at least one hour.

9oz/250g dried beans (mixed or single-variety) or 1.1lb/500g cooked beans from a jar or BPA-free tin

7oz/200g top-quality sardines in olive oil from a jar or BPA-free tin

1 small red onion, finely chopped

1 clove garlic, crushed

1 rib celery, finely cubed

½ red pepper, finely cubed

2 tbsp parsley, chopped

grated zest of ½ lemon

10 black olives or 10 capers (rinsed), coarsely chopped

6fl oz/¾ cup/180ml Italian dressing (p. 234)

salt & freshly ground black pepper

Omega express

1 large or 2 medium beets (about 15oz/400g), cooked and peeled (you can use ready-cooked vacuum-packed beets)

15oz/400g arugula, lamb's lettuce or other salad greens

4-5 tbsp Italian dressing (p. 234), perhaps including some walnut oil

7oz/200g whole sardines in olive oil from a jar or BPA-free tin, drained and coarsely broken up

3.5oz/¾ cup/100g walnuts, coarsely chopped

This salad's many merits include speed of preparation (you can throw it together in less than 10 minutes if you keep a supply of salad dressing in your refrigerator), a plethora of anti-cancer ingredients, the esthetic appeal of ruby-red beets nestling among bright-green leaves; and of course, its utter deliciousness! Serves 4 as an *hors d'oeuvre*.

Cut the beets into roughly ½-inch (1cm) cubes, place in a bowl and drizzle with 2 tablespoons of the dressing; leave to infuse while you prepare the rest of the salad. (If you do this ahead of time, the beets will absorb more of the garlicky-lemony flavors and taste even better. A tub of marinating beet cubes keeps in the refrigerator for about five days.)

Lightly dress salad leaves with the remaining vinaigrette and arrange on serving plates or in a large, flat salad bowl. Scatter with beet cubes, sardine chunks and walnuts and serve.

Variation

This also tastes delicious if you substitute sardines with fresh goats' cheese or ewes' milk feta cheese – though this means you'll get fewer omega-3 fats.

Greek salad – a timeless classic

This crunchy, fresh and fragrant salad is a Mediterranean summer classic. Enjoy it on its own as an appetizer or as an accompaniment to grilled fish, chicken or legumes.

In a bowl, combine all the salad vegetables and herbs. Just before serving, drizzle with the dressing and toss lightly. Garnish with feta cheese and olives.

1 head crisp lettuce, coarsely shredded
3-4 spring onions, thinly sliced
2oz/50g black pitted olives
4oz/100g cherry tomatoes, halved
1 cucumber, cubed
2 tbsp chopped fresh mint
1 tbsp fresh oregano
7oz/200g feta cheese, cubed
4-5 tbsp Italian dressing (p. 234)

Avocado, apple and walnut salad

This unusual salad combining fruits and vegetables is surprisingly tasty, quick and easy to make and can be enjoyed all year round. Meltingly soft avocadoes, crunchy nuts and crisp celery and apples create exciting textural sensations, while the sweet-and-salty flavor contrasts keep your taste buds on their toes. A sure hit with young and old.

In a small serving bowl, combine apples, celery and avocados, and sprinkle with chopped parsley, cranberries and walnuts. In a small mixing bowl, lightly whisk oils, lemon juice and acacia honey. Pour over cubed fruits and vegetables, toss lightly and serve immediately.

This salad can be served as an appetizer on individual plates, garnished with a few leaves of arugula or other salad greens.

1 apple, cored and cubed
1 rib celery, cubed
2 ripe avocados, peeled and cubed
2 tbsp chopped parsley
1 tbsp dried cranberries
1 tbsp walnuts, chopped
1 tbsp walnut oil
1 tbsp olive oil
1 tbsp lemon juice
1 tsp acacia honey
salt & pepper

Golden quinoa tabouleh

9oz/heaped 1 cup/250g dry quinoa, rinsed and drained

1pint/2 cups/500ml water

½ vegetable bouillon cube

1 tsp turmeric

3 tbsp olive oil

2 tbsp lemon juice

pinch of freshly grated lemon zest

2 cloves garlic, crushed

½ tsp ras el hanout (Moroccan specialty spice mix; see p. 183), or a pinch each of turmeric, ground coriander, ginger, cumin and paprika powder

½ tsp cinnamon

9oz/250g finely cubed tomatoes

2 spring onions, finely chopped

2 heaped tbsp coarsely chopped mint

2oz/50g coarsely chopped parsley

salt & freshly ground black pepper

Tabouleh is a delicious Middle Eastern salad of cracked wheat with finely cubed tomatoes, cucumbers, onions, spices and oodles of chopped parsley. Here, I have replaced cracked wheat with the less-glycemic quinoa, whose delicious crunchy texture and nutty flavor match the other ingredients perfectly. Serves 4.

Place rinsed quinoa in a medium pot and cover with water; add stock cube and turmeric and bring to the boil. Cover and simmer on low heat until the grains are al dente. Remove from heat and tip into a wide bowl to cool for about 20 minutes.

In a large bowl, combine oil, lemon juice and zest, crushed garlic and spices. Tip cooled quinoa into the bowl, add chopped tomatoes, onions and herbs and toss gently. Season to taste with lemon juice, salt and pepper. Chill until serving.

Eggplant caviar

Enjoy this creamy eggplant mousse as a dip for carrot sticks, celery ribs, radishes or raw pepper strips, spread it onto a slice of crisply toasted whole grain sourdough bread or slather it onto a perfectly ripe avocado. Smear it onto cucumber slices, canapé-style. Or stuff it into salad-leaf rolls for wonderfully messy finger-food. The possibilities are endless! Serves 4 as an *hors d'oeuvre* or an accompaniment to a main dish.

4 medium eggplants

3 tbsp flat-leaf parsley, roughly chopped

1-2 cloves garlic, crushed

4 tbsp extra virgin olive oil

squeeze of lemon juice

salt & freshly ground black pepper

Heat the grill to its highest setting. Prick eggplants several times with the tip of a sharp knife to prevent them bursting. Line a baking tray with baking parchment, place the eggplants on it and slide under hot grill. Turn the eggplants by a quarter rotation whenever the skin starts to blister.

After 20-25 minutes, the eggplants should be dark and blistered outside and soft inside. Remove from grill and cool for 10 minutes. Cut off the stalks and slice eggplants in half. Scrape the soft flesh out of the skin and into a sieve; drain for a few minutes.

Place chopped parsley, crushed garlic and olive oil in a mixing bowl. Add drained eggplant flesh and mix with a fork, making light cutting or chopping movements to break down the eggplant. If you like a very creamy puree, give it a few short bursts with a handheld blender. Season to taste with salt, pepper and lemon juice.

Variations
- Cubed tomatoes and a finely chopped red onion can be added just before serving for extra crunch and flavor.
- Two chopped hard-boiled eggs scattered over this dish just before serving boost this dish's protein content.
- Instead of parsley, you can use chopped mint or cilantro.
- A tablespoon of sesame paste (*tahini*) will turn this into the Lebanese delicacy *baba ghanoush*.

Red cabbage and walnut slaw

1 shallot, finely chopped

2 tbsp apple cider or red wine vinegar

2 tbsp walnut oil

2 tbsp olive oil

½ red cabbage, quartered, cored and finely sliced by hand or food processor

1 large apple (peeled if non-organic), finely grated

2 tbsp raisins

2oz/50g walnuts, coarsely chopped

salt, pepper

A crunchy, fruity and dramatically colored salad for those dreary winter months – this makes a pleasant (and lighter) change from traditional coleslaw with mayonnaise.

In a salad bowl, combine chopped shallot and vinegar and leave to infuse five minutes. Then add oil, salt and pepper. Add shredded cabbage, grated apple and raisins and toss with dressing; if you have time, leave to infuse for ½ hour. Sprinkle with walnuts and serve.

Fennel and orange winter salad

Crunchy, fresh and super-quick to prepare – just what you want when the days are short, energy levels are low and you want something zingy to lift you out of your wintery torpor.

If segmenting oranges (explained below) sounds too fiddly, simply peel the oranges carefully, separate the segments with your fingers and cut each segment into 4-5 chunks; if the orange is juicy and tasty, no one will mind eating a bit of pith; it's extra fiber and a source of anti-cancer nutrients! Serves 4.

2 bulbs fennel (choose smaller bulbs – they're less stringy)

2 juicy oranges

2 tbsp best-quality olive oil

1 tbsp chopped parsley, cilantro or fennel greens

salt & freshly ground black pepper

Cut stalks off fennel bulbs, reserving the fronds if they haven't wilted. Slice the hard, brown bases off the fennel, cut bulbs in half and remove hard cores. Slice as thinly as possible and place in a salad bowl.

Next, using a small, sharp knife, segment the orange on a plate, to catch the juice. Cut the top and bottom off of the orange so it can stand flat on the plate. Stand the orange on one end and, with small sawing movements, cut down the side to peel the orange, following the curve of the orange downwards. Remove as much of the white membrane as you can.

Next, cut the orange segments between the membranes and lift each segment out carefully. Squeeze out any juice from the remaining peel, adding this to salad bowl along with any juices that may have escaped as you were preparing the orange.

Drizzle with olive oil, season with salt and pepper and toss lightly. Sprinkle with chopped parsley, cilantro or fennel greens.

Variation

This is equally delicious using endives; the sweet oranges and bitter endives offset each other beautifully. Replace fennel bulbs with 2-3 endives, remove cores, halve and slice into ½ inch/1 cm slices. This tastes good sprinkled with lightly toasted, chopped walnuts, too.

Grilled goats' cheese salad

2 apples, peeled if not organic

1 fresh goats' cheese log (approx. 7oz/200g) cut into 8 equal slices

mixed salad greens (lettuce, arugula, radicchio, endive, etc.)

seasonal salad vegetables of your choice, such as tomatoes, avocados, grated beets or carrots, peas, cooked fava beans, steamed asparagus

4 tbsp nuts (pine nuts, hazelnuts, walnuts)

seasonal fruit according to taste: dried raisins, cranberries, apricots (cubed); or fresh grapes, apples, pears (cubed)

2 tsp honey (optional)

pinch of herbes de Provence or paprika powder

3fl oz/¹/₃ cup/80ml Classic French Vinaigrette (p. 234)

A French bistro classic, this bright mixed salad adorned with melting goats' cheese croutons never fails to delight. Here I've replaced the habitual white-bread croutons with slices of apple, which lend a fruity note.

Apart from the lettuce leaves and cheese croutons, there are no fixed ingredients for this salad, so use whatever's in season. In spring peas, fava beans or asparagus, topped with toasted hazelnuts and hazelnut vinaigrette, are delicious. In summer, tomatoes, avocados, sweet onions and cucumber, topped with toasted pine nuts, are tasty. During fall and winter, root vegetables (raw grated beet or carrot), dried fruit (raisins or cranberries), endive or radicchio leaves and walnuts are lovely. Serves 4.

Preheat grill on high setting.

Wash and dry all vegetables and fruits. Cut each apple into 4 slices of about ¼ inch (6mm) each yielding 8 slices in total and lay these onto a baking tray. Place goats' cheese rounds on apple slices.

Combine salad greens in a wide serving bowl, toss lightly with salad dressing. Heap these onto serving plates or leave in the bowl.

Place baking tray beneath grill and watch closely; the goats' cheese should begin bubbling slightly but shouldn't start melting, or it will run off the apples!

Scatter dried or fresh fruit and nuts over salad. Place apple-and-goats'-cheese croutons on top of salad. If you wish, you can drizzle each crouton with a few drops of honey and *herbes de Provence* or a sprinkling of paprika powder. Serve immediately.

Niçoise salad

There are almost as many versions of this famous salad as there are cooks. The classic version usually includes black olives, fava beans, cucumbers, tomatoes, raw bell peppers, hard-boiled eggs and anchovies. Feel free to add any other Mediterranean vegetables such as fennel, avocado or roasted sweet peppers. This recipe makes a light lunch for four; if you like, you can serve it as an *hors d'oeuvre* topped with just a few anchovies from a jar instead of the freshly cooked fish. Serves 4 as a light main course.

In a large pot, steam the green beans until *al dente* (about 3-4 minutes for frozen beans, 5-6 minutes for fresh – depending on thickness). Strain and rinse with cold water to preserve their bright green color. Set aside.

On a serving platter, arrange lettuce, beans, fennel, onion, tomatoes, olives, peppers and whatever other vegetables you may be using and drizzle with half the dressing.

Heat 1 tbsp olive oil in a pan and cook fish for 1-2 minutes on each side. Place fish and egg quarters atop the greens and pour over the remaining dressing. Serve immediately.

11oz/300g green beans (fresh or frozen)

medium head of romaine lettuce, chopped, or mixed salad greens (about 15oz/400g)

1 fennel bulb, halved, cored and finely sliced

1 spring onion or shallot, finely chopped

12 ripe cherry tomatoes, halved, or 3 large tomatoes, coarsely cubed

about 16 pitted black olives, sliced

1 red bell pepper, de-seeded, quartered and finely sliced

1 tbsp olive oil

6-8 fresh mackerel fillets or 12-16 fresh sardine fillets (depending on size)

2 hard-boiled eggs, cooled, peeled and quartered

4-5 tbsp Classic French vinaigrette (p. 234)

Sauerkraut and apple salad

7 oz/200 g raw
sauerkraut

2 firm apples, finely
grated

1 tbsp olive oil

2 tbsp walnut oil

1 tbsp acacia honey

few drops of lemon juice

3 tbsp nuts (hazelnuts,
walnuts and pecans
are particularly tasty),
coarsely chopped

5-6 dried apricots, cut
into small pieces with
kitchen scissors

Naturally fermented, uncooked sauerkraut – available in most health food stores – is an excellent source of essential nutrients, beneficial bacteria that are so important for digestive health, and a generous helping of fiber. Raw sauerkraut is rather tart on its own, but combined, as here, with grated apple, dried fruit and nuts and a hint of honey, it makes a delicious, quick and easy salad. Plain, raw sauerkraut keeps for weeks in the refrigerator, so try to eat some on most days during the cabbage season – it may help ward off some winter bugs. Serves 4.

Place sauerkraut in a mixing bowl and grate apples on top with a hand-held box grater.

In a separate small bowl, combine oils, honey and lemon juice and drizzle dressing over cabbage-apple mix.

Using a spoon and fork, toss the vegetables and the dressing thoroughly until the sauerkraut is untangled and the mixture is evenly combined.

Sprinkle with chopped nuts and apricots and serve.

Summery sardine salad

This salad tastes like a summer's sea breeze. It's best made with fresh runner beans and tomatoes, but it's almost as good in winter with frozen beans and sun-dried tomatoes. This can be enjoyed as an *hors d'oeuvre* or light lunch. Serves 4.

In a small pot, boil the eggs for 10 minutes. Rinse under cold water and set aside; once cool enough to handle, peel and quarter.

While the eggs are boiling, toast pine nuts in a dry skillet on low heat, stirring constantly until they turn golden and release their nutty fragrance (2-3 minutes).

Meanwhile, steam green beans until *al dente* (3-4 minutes). Strain and rinse thoroughly with cold water so they preserve their vibrant green color.

Cube tomatoes and cut hard-boiled eggs into quarters. Coarsely chop parsley.

In a large serving bowl, toss beans with dressing and chopped parsley. Scatter tomatoes over the beans followed by the egg quarters.

In a large skillet on medium heat, warm olive oil. Dredge sardines lightly in flour and cook in the pan on medium heat for 2 minutes on each side. Remove and place atop the salad. Sprinkle with pine nuts and serve.

Variations
Fresh sardines can be replaced with sardines from a jar or can; these don't need to be cooked, thus cutting down preparation time.

---

4 eggs

4 tbsp pine nuts

1¼ lb/600 g green beans, topped & tailed

7 oz/200 g tomatoes, cubed

2 tbsp coarsely chopped parsley

3 tbsp olive oil

3 tbsp whole spelt, wheat or corn flour

11oz/300g fresh sardine fillets

4-5 tbsp Italian dressing (p. 234)

Soups and stews

Soups and stews are quintessentially Mediterranean dishes; to this day, the evening meal in France is called *le souper* and in many French homes people eat soup for dinner.

The soup section in this book is rather extensive. This is because soups have so many advantages: they are easy to make in relatively little time, they can be cooked in advance and stored easily in a refrigerator or freezer for re-heating, and they make it easy for people to increase their vegetable intake.

Soups are also wonderful convalescent food as cooking and pureeing makes them easier to eat, digest and assimilate. Thick, nourishing soups can be eaten as light stand-alone meals; if you want to serve them as *hors d'oeuvres*, simply serve smaller portions and freeze the rest.

None of the soups in this book require complicated procedures. While home-made stock tastes wonderful and is very nourishing, most of us don't have the time to make it. Instead of the "real thing" it's fine to use bouillon cubes, although you should try to buy bouillon cubes without chemical flavor enhancers like monosodium glutamate. Many supermarkets also sell delicious chicken or vegetable stock in bottles or cartons.

Having said this, if ever you're left with a roast-chicken carcass, pop it in a pot, cover it with water, add a chopped carrot, an onion, a celery rib, a leek, a bay leaf and a sprig of thyme, simmer for two hours and drain through a fine sieve. You'll get fantastic chicken stock that you can use straight away or freeze for later.

As with salads, you can sprinkle a variety of garnishes over soups to add visual and textural interest. They might include toasted, chopped nuts or seeds, sprouted grains or seeds, a grating of parmesan, a drizzle of Cashew cream (p. 231), some cubes of avocado or cooked beet, a swirl of herb *coulis*, a few drops of a particularly aromatic olive or walnut oil – the possibilities are endless.

While cream in soups is delicious, it doesn't agree with everyone. That's why I often use Cashew cream as an alternative to dairy cream. It looks and tastes very similar to dairy cream and has the added advantage of thickening sauces in a manner similar to corn starch. It's quick and easy to make yourself – all you need is a small, powerful blender. You will notice that I use it frequently in this book; if you don't like it, it can be replaced with ordinary cream or *crème fraiche* (ideally organic).

Vegetable soup for beginners

If you are new to cooking, this dish allows you to enjoy a satisfying and nutrient-dense meal requiring minimal skills and time. The recipe includes some very basic vegetables, but you can vary the list in accordance with the seasons and your mood. A few cubes of left-over cooked chicken meat or marinated tofu can provide a tasty protein boost. You can serve this chunky or pureed, or puree half and combine the two. The clove of garlic added just before serving will add pungency; if you don't like fresh garlic, add it at the beginning of the recipe. Serves 4.

In a large, heavy cooking pot, warm 1 tablespoon olive oil on medium heat and add chopped onion, 1 clove garlic, carrots and leeks. Cook, stirring, for 5 minutes; then add beans, hot stock, thyme and bay leaf. Cover and simmer on low heat for 10 minutes, or until carrots are soft.

Add chopped broccoli and cook for another 5 minutes. Squeeze second clove of garlic into the soup with a garlic press.

Remove bay leaf, transfer some or all of the soup to a blender and puree until you have the desired consistency. Sprinkle with chopped parsley, season to taste with salt, pepper and lemon juice and serve. Drizzle a little olive oil over the soup for added flavor.

1 tbsp olive oil, plus some more for drizzling

1 large onion, chopped

2 cloves garlic, crushed

2 large carrots, peeled and finely cubed

2 leeks, cleaned and finely sliced (including half the green sections)

4oz/100g navy beans, pre-cooked or from a jar (drained and rinsed)

2 pints/1l hot vegetable or chicken stock

1 generous pinch thyme

1 bay leaf

1 small head broccoli, coarsely chopped

2 tbsp chopped parsley

drizzle of lemon juice

salt & freshly ground black pepper

Broccoli soup

2 tbsp olive oil

1 small onion, finely chopped

1 rib celery, finely chopped

1 clove garlic, finely chopped

1 large head broccoli, coarsely chopped (including the stalk)

1 bay leaf

1 pinch thyme

1½ pints/3 cups/750 ml chicken or vegetable stock

4 tbsp Cashew cream (p. 231)

salt & freshly ground black pepper

lemon juice

red pepper flakes or paprika powder

This is one of the quickest and most satisfying soups imaginable. Don't overcook the broccoli – it can go from a luscious bright green to a murky khaki-brown in the space of a minute! Delicious served with spicy Cashew cream (p. 231) or Avocado-Blue cheese cream (p. 232). Serves 4.

In a heavy cooking pot on medium heat, warm the olive oil and sweat onion, celery and garlic for 4-5 minutes until the onion is translucent. Add broccoli, herbs and stock, bring to the boil, reduce heat, cover and cook for 6-7 minutes.

When the broccoli is soft but *al dente*, remove from heat, take out bay leaf and transfer vegetables and stock to blender. Blend into a creamy puree (in two batches if your blender is small); add hot water to dilute if necessary.

Season to taste with pepper, salt and lemon juice. Serve in individual bowls with a swirl of Cashew cream and a sprinkling of red pepper flakes or paprika powder.

Cream of cauliflower soup

Here, cauliflower is paired with curry and turmeric to produce a comforting yet invigoratingly spicy and brightly colored soup. A boon for the tired cook, it takes a mere 20 minutes to prepare and makes a deliciously filling, yet light, supper. Serves 4.

In a heavy cooking pot, gently warm olive oil, add onion, ginger and garlic and cook for 4-5 minutes, stirring constantly, until the onions are translucent. Add spices and keep stirring for another 1-2 minutes until a nutty, toasty aroma develops; take care not to burn the spices or they will taste bitter.

Add chopped cauliflower and stir until well coated with the spices. Add stock and gently bring to the boil. Lower the temperature and simmer, covered, for 10 minutes. Once the cauliflower is soft, liquidize vegetables and their broth in a blender, add coconut milk and season to taste with salt, pepper and lemon juice.

Garnish with chopped hazelnuts, parsley or cilantro and serve immediately.

2 tbsp olive oil

1 large onion, chopped

2 cloves garlic, finely chopped

1 tbsp finely grated fresh ginger

1 tsp ground turmeric

1 tsp curry powder

1 small cauliflower, coarsely chopped

1½ pints/3 cups/750 ml vegetable or chicken stock

2fl oz/¼ cup/60ml coconut milk

squeeze of lemon juice

handful of hazelnuts, lightly toasted and coarsely chopped

2 tbsp chopped cilantro or parsley

salt & freshly ground black pepper

Green-tea chicken soup

1 small chicken (2-3lb/1-1½ kg), any giblets removed

4 large leeks

8 medium carrots, peeled

1 yellow onion

4 ribs celery

1 large chunk of fresh ginger root (1-1½ inch/3-4 cm), coarsely sliced

1 tsp thyme

2 bay leaves

10fl oz/1 ¼ cups/300ml strong green tea

3.5oz/⅔ cup/100g green peas (fresh or frozen)

squirt of lemon juice

3 tbsp chopped parsley

salt & freshly ground black pepper

Chicken soup is a very forgiving dish: no matter how much you play around with ingredients and seasonings, it usually comes out rich and comforting. This recipe doesn't actually involve much work; just some vegetable scrubbing, peeling, chopping and patience as the chicken, vegetables and herbs yield their comforting aromas to the broth and to your home! Serves 6.

Wash the chicken and place in a large cooking pot with a lid.

Cut the dark green ends off the leeks and rinse under running water to remove any grit; coarsely chop 2 leeks, setting the other 2 aside. Coarsely chop 4 carrots, the onion, 2 celery ribs and the ginger. Tuck these around the chicken in the pot along with the bay leaves and thyme. Fill the pot with just enough cold water to barely cover the chicken. Bring to the boil, skim off any foam that may rise to the surface, cover and simmer on lowest heat for 1½ hours.

While the chicken is cooking, peel remaining carrots, quarter lengthwise and cube. Finely cube the remaining celery ribs and thinly slice the whites of the remaining leeks. When the chicken is cooked through, lift it out of the stock and set aside to cool on a plate. Pour the broth through a fine-meshed strainer or cotton cloth into another large pot and discard the first batch of vegetables.

Bring chicken broth to the boil again and add finely chopped vegetables: first the carrots and celery, 5 minutes later the leeks. Cook for another 5 minutes, or until the vegetables are tender but *al dente*.

While the vegetables are cooking, remove chicken skin and discard. Shred the meat and set aside.

When the vegetables are soft, add green tea, shredded meat and peas and reheat gently for 2-3 minutes. Season with pepper, salt and lemon juice. Sprinkle with parsley and serve.

Watercress soup with poached eggs

This nourishing soup is a tasty way of getting watercress – an under-appreciated member of the Brassica family – into your diet. The egg provides extra protein, making this meal suitable for a light lunch. If you can't find watercress, replace it with arugula (sold in the salad section of many grocery stores) or spinach. Serves 4.

In a heavy cooking pot sweat lightly salted leeks in the olive oil for 5 minutes; add chestnuts or potatoes, whichever using, cover and cook on low heat for 10 minutes, stirring occasionally and checking that nothing gets stuck to the base of the pot. If it does, add a little water.

Add watercress and stock and bring to the boil. Cook for 6-8 minutes until the vegetables are soft. Pour into blender and liquidize to the desired consistency. Pour back into the pot, season with salt, pepper and lemon juice, cover and set aside.

In another large pot, heat water about 2 inches/4 cm deep. Once it boils, add a large pinch of salt and the vinegar and lower the heat to keep the water at a low, rolling boil. Lightly grease a ladle and break an egg into it. Hold the ladle close to the surface of the water, gently tilt and slide the egg into the water against the side of the pot. If the eggs are fresh, the white will remain neatly wrapped around the yolk.

Repeat swiftly with the remaining eggs. Remember in which order you put them into the water as you will need to retrieve them in the same order. Cook 2 minutes for a runny yolk or 3 minutes for a firmer yolk. Remove each egg with a slotted spoon, rinse briefly under cold water to halt the cooking and place on a plate until all eggs have been removed.

Reheat the soup, ladle into soup plates, place a poached egg at the center of each plate, garnish with watercress leaves and red pepper flakes and serve immediately.

2 tbsp olive oil

3 leeks (white parts only), thoroughly cleaned and thinly sliced

3.5 oz/100 g chestnuts (cooked and vacuum-packed) or 3 small new potatoes

2 bunches of watercress (15oz/400g total), stems removed and coarsely chopped (save a few leaves for garnish)

1½ pint/750ml chicken or vegetable stock

salt & freshly ground black pepper

few drops of lemon juice

4 very fresh eggs at room temperature

3 tbsp white-wine vinegar

pinch of red pepper flakes

Moroccan chicken & garbanzo stew

3 tbsp olive oil

1.1lb/500g chicken leg portions

2 large onions, chopped

1 rib celery, cubed

3 cloves garlic

1 tbsp freshly grated or dried, ground ginger

1 tsp turmeric

1 tsp ground coriander

½ tsp ground cumin

½ tsp paprika powder

pinch of saffron

1 cinnamon stick

pinch of chili powder

2 pints/1l chicken stock

7oz/200g cubed pumpkin or carrots

15oz/400g cooked garbanzos, drained

15oz/400g cubed tomatoes (fresh or from a jar)

zest and juice of ½ lemon

3 tbsp chopped cilantro

salt & freshly ground black pepper

This well-known dish (called *chorba* in Arabic) is a nourishing North African stew often eaten just before sunrise during Ramadan, the Islamic month of fasting. As with so many Mediterranean stews, there are as many versions of *chorba* as there are cooks – some prepared with lamb, others with veal, some containing vermicelli noodles, others potatoes. Feel free to add other vegetables, such as green beans, chopped fresh spinach, turnips or zucchini, depending on the season and on your mood. However, the garbanzos should remain as they give the soup bulk and bite; if you like, you can replace the chicken with small cubes of firm tofu. Serves 4.

In a large, heavy cooking pot, warm 1 tablespoon olive oil and cook the chicken portions on gentle heat until golden on both sides. Remove and set aside.

Add remaining olive oil and cook onion, celery and garlic until the onions are translucent. Add ginger and spices and cook for another minute, stirring to prevent the spices burning. Add stock and carrots or pumpkin, and bring to the boil.

Return chicken portions to the pot, add garbanzos and bring back to the boil; then reduce heat and simmer on low heat for 20 minutes. Add tomatoes and continue cooking for 15-20 minutes, until the vegetables are soft and the chicken is cooked through. Remove chicken, discard skin, shred into bite-sized pieces and return to stew to reheat.

Season to taste with lemon zest and juice, salt and pepper and sprinkle with chopped cilantro leaves.

Coconut lentil stew & avocado relish

This chunky stew is a combination of classically Mediterranean ingredients – onions, garlic, lentils and tomatoes – enriched with the exotic aromas of ginger, turmeric, coriander and coconut. A dollop of avocado relish (p. 152) at the end adds a burst of color and freshness to this spicy, warming stew. Additional vegetables such as finely chopped carrots, leeks, celery, pumpkin, peas, green beans or fresh spinach work well here, as does finely cubed tofu or chicken for added protein. Serves 4.

In a heavy cooking pot, gently warm olive or coconut oil and cook onion, garlic and ginger, stirring frequently, for 4-5 minutes. Add spices and continue cooking and stirring for another minute, taking care not to burn the spices.

Add lentils, bay leaf and water, bring to the boil, cover and simmer on low heat for 30-40 minutes (15 minutes if using precooked lentils). If using tofu or chicken, add at this stage. Vegetables like carrots, green beans, leeks or celery should also be added now. Stir occasionally and check there's enough water so the lentils don't stick to the bottom of the pan.

While the soup is simmering prepare avocado relish (p. 152).

When the lentils are tender, add tomatoes and cook for another 10 minutes. Finally, add coconut milk and stir gently, allowing it to warm through but not boil. Add lemon zest and season with salt and pepper. Serve avocado relish alongside the soup.

2 tbsp olive oil or coconut oil

1 large onion, coarsely chopped

2 cloves garlic, crushed

1 inch/2cm ginger, finely grated

1 heaped tsp turmeric

1 heaped tsp ground coriander

1 level tsp cumin

1 level tsp cardamom

1 bay leaf

9oz/1¼ cup/250g dry French green lentils (or 18oz/2½ cups/500g pre-cooked lentils)

2 pints/1l water (if using precooked lentils, use 1 pint/500ml)

15oz/400g coarsely cubed tomatoes (fresh or from a jar)

10fl oz/1¼ cup/300ml pure coconut milk

zest of ½ lemon, finely grated

1 portion avocado relish (p. 152)

Spicy beet and coconut soup

1 tbsp olive or coconut oil

1 small onion, finely chopped

3 cloves garlic, crushed

1 tbsp finely grated fresh ginger

1 tsp curry powder

1.1lb/500g beets (cooked and vacuum-packed), coarsely cubed

13½ fl oz/1⅔ cups/400ml chicken or vegetable stock

10oz/300ml coconut milk

1 tbsp balsamic vinegar

salt & freshly ground black pepper to taste

4 tsp Cashew cream (p. 231) or coconut cream

sprigs of herbs such as cilantro, parsley or chervil.

Although most people know that beets are a super-food, many of us just can't get past their earthy taste. In this velvety, vibrant soup – which can be enjoyed hot or cold – ginger, garlic, curry and creamy coconut milk transform the much-maligned purple root into an elegant and refreshing delicacy that will leave you wishing you'd made twice as much! Serves 4.

Heat oil in a medium pot and gently cook chopped onions for 4-5 minutes, until translucent. Add ginger, garlic and curry powder and continue cooking for another minute, stirring frequently.

Add beets and stock and simmer for 10 minutes, then remove from heat.

Transfer to a blender and liquidize until you obtain a velvety-smooth puree. Return to the pot. Add coconut milk and season with balsamic vinegar, salt and pepper to taste. Try to balance the beets' sweetness, the curry's heat, the vinegar's acidity and the salt's saltiness (see FASSU – p. 112). Keep tasting – you'll know when it's right.

If you are serving this soup hot, re-heat it on very gentle heat; ladle into soup bowls and garnish with a sprig of herbs and a swirl of Cashew or coconut cream. If serving cold, chill soup for 3 hours. Then ladle into glasses or cups and add cream and herbs just before serving.

Gascon garlic soup

This is the nourishing south-western French soup described on p. 32 (*Tourin à l'ail*). Despite its high garlic content, it tastes sweet, creamy and utterly comforting. Thick hunks of wholegrain bread – *pain de campagne* – are sometimes used to bulk up the soup. When doing this, place a slice or two of bread at the bottom of the soup tureen, pour soup on top and let the bread soften for a few minutes before serving. Serves 4.

In a heavy cooking pot, heat olive oil and add onion and garlic; cook until translucent. Add stock and cook for 15 minutes. Pour into a liquidizer and blend into a velvety soup. Return to pot on low heat.

Separate eggs into two bowls and beat whites with a fork; then slowly pour whites into the soup while stirring with a balloon whisk and remove from heat as soon as they form fine threads.

In the other bowl, combine the yolks with vinegar; add some of the hot soup and mix. Now pour the yolks into the soup and stir gently until all ingredients are combined. Re-heat gently but do not bring back to the boil.

Season with salt and pepper and serve.

---

2 tbsp olive oil

1 onion, peeled and finely sliced

2 bulbs garlic, cloves peeled and coarsely chopped

2 pints/1l stock (chicken or vegetable)

3 large eggs

1 tbsp red wine vinegar

salt & freshly ground black pepper

Cream of mushroom soup

½ to 1 oz/10-15g dried porcini or mixed mushrooms

2 tbsp olive oil

2 large shallots, or 1 small onion, finely chopped

4 whole fresh shiitake mushrooms

15oz/400g fresh mushrooms, coarsely chopped

½ tsp thyme

6 cooked chestnuts (from a jar or vacuum-packed) or 1 tbsp whole grain spelt or wheat flour (optional)

2fl oz/¼ cup/60ml white wine

2 pints/1l vegetable broth

squeeze of lemon juice

salt & freshly ground black pepper

2 tbsp finely chopped parsley

4 tbsp Cashew cream (p. 231)

pinch of red pepper flakes or paprika powder

The concentrated flavors of this soup belie its speed of preparation. You can use any mushrooms, but those with the greatest immune-boosting virtues include shiitake, oyster, porcini or chestnut mushrooms. Some people like their mushroom soup light, with small bits of mushroom floating in the aromatic broth. If you prefer a thicker soup, throw in a few pre-cooked chestnuts or add a little flour. Serves 4.

Place dried mushrooms in a bowl and cover with hot water; rehydrate for 15 minutes.

In a heavy cooking pot on low heat, gently warm oil and cook the shallots for 3-4 minutes until translucent. Add the fresh mushrooms and thyme and cook for another 4-5 minutes until the mushrooms are soft and releasing their juices. (For a thicker soup, add flour or chestnuts now; if using flour, stir well until vegetables are evenly coated.)

With a slotted spoon, remove rehydrated mushrooms from their soaking water, chop coarsely and add to mushroom-shallot mix. Add white wine and vegetable broth. Strain mushroom-soaking water through a cheesecloth to remove any forest grit and add to the mushrooms. Simmer for another 15 minutes.

With a ladle, transfer soup to a blender in two batches; for a slightly chunky soup, blend the first batch to a fine, creamy texture and the second batch only briefly to preserve some chunks; combine in the cooking pot. Season to taste with salt, pepper and lemon juice.

Ladle soup into serving bowls, drizzle with Cashew cream and sprinkle with red pepper flakes and chopped parsley.

French onion soup

This French bistro classic is a real crowd pleaser, and so easy to make! Red onions and wine produce a deep-purple soup that beautifully offsets the cheese crouton. If you can't find red onions, this also works well with white ones. This filling soup can constitute a light dinner, or you can serve smaller quantities as an *hors d'oeuvre*. Asking you to slice the onions by hand may seem unnecessarily sadistic and of course you can use a food processor if you prefer. It's just that machine-sliced onions turn slushy when cooked in a way that hand-cut ones don't. Serves 4 as a main dish or 6 as an *hors d'oeuvre*.

In a large pot, warm olive oil and cook onions, sprinkled with a generous pinch of salt, for 10-15 minutes until they start to brown, stirring steadily. Add wine, garlic and herbs and continue cooking on medium heat for five minutes. Now add stock, stir and bring to boil.

Simmer, covered, for 30-40 minutes until the onions are soft and the soup has darkened. Season with vinegar, salt and pepper. Cover and remove from heat.

To prepare croutons, place bread slices on a baking tray and toast on one side under a hot grill until golden. Remove baking tray, turn bread over and sprinkle evenly with grated cheese. Return to grill and toast until the cheese has melted.

Ladle soup into individual soup bowls. Remove baking tray from oven and use a spatula to lift up the hot croutons and slide them onto each bowl of soup, where they will soak up the aromatic broth and soften.

2 tbsp olive oil

2.2lb/1kg red onions, peeled and sliced

1-2 cloves garlic, finely chopped

4fl oz/½ cup/120ml red wine

½ tsp thyme

2 bay leaves

1 chicken or beef bouillon (organic) dissolved in 2 pints/1l water

1 tbsp red-wine vinegar

salt & freshly ground black pepper

1 small slice whole grain sourdough bread per person

4-5 tbsp grated cheese (e.g., ewes' or goats' milk cheddar)

Curried pumpkin and apple soup & toasted pumpkin seeds

2 tbsp olive or coconut oil

1 large onion, chopped

1 tbsp grated fresh ginger

1½ lb/750g Hokkaido or butternut squash or pumpkin, peeled and cubed

1 tsp curry powder

1 tsp turmeric

1¼ pints/750ml vegetable stock

11oz/300g apples, cored and cubed

7fl oz/scant 1 cup/200ml coconut milk

squeeze of lemon juice

chives for garnish

salt & freshly ground black pepper

4 tsp Cashew cream (p. 231) or toasted pumpkin oil

Tamari-toasted pumpkin seeds

4 tbsp raw pumpkin seeds

1 tsp tamari (wheat-free soy sauce)

This thick, warming soup makes a comforting fall or winter meal packed with nutrients. To counterbalance the vegetables' natural sweetness, you can add a few drops of chili sauce. Chop all vegetables into fairly small pieces; this way they will cook faster and retain maximum vitamin content. Serves 4-6.

Heat oil in a large, heavy-bottomed pan, add onion and cook on medium heat until soft. Add grated ginger and cook another 2 minutes. Add squash, curry powder and turmeric and cook with the onion, stirring constantly, for another 1-2 minutes, then pour in stock. Cover and simmer on low heat for 10 minutes. Add apples, cover and cook for another 10-15 minutes until squash and apples are soft.

While the soup is cooking, toast pumpkin seeds in a dry skillet, stirring with a wooden spoon until they start to puff up and crackle (3-4 minutes). Add tamari; there will be much hissing and steam but keep stirring and soon the pan will be dry and the seeds coated with a delicious salty crust. Tip onto a plate to cool.

When squash and apples are soft, transfer to blender and puree to a fine consistency. When fully blended, pour into a clean pot. Add coconut milk, reheat and season to taste with salt, pepper and lemon juice. Remove from heat and cover.

Ladle soup into bowls and dress each portion with a teaspoon of Cashew cream (p. 231) or toasted pumpkin oil. Sprinkle with pumpkin seeds and chives for garnish.

Provençal *pistou* soup

The line separating French and Italian cooking is often a fine one, as this delicious Provençal vegetable soup - which closely resembles Italy's *minestrone* - shows. The difference between the two is that *soupe au pistou* uses summer vegetables such as zucchini, tomatoes and green beans, rather than the more wintery carrots, leeks and celery that form the basis of minestrone. By adding *pistou* just before serving you can create a veritable taste sensation. *Pistou* is a fragrant combination of basil, olive oil and garlic that closely resembles Italy's pesto, only without the pine nuts and Parmesan cheese. If you can't get hold of fresh basil, just add a dollop of premium-quality shop-bought pesto. Serves 4.

In a heavy cooking pot, warm olive oil and cook chopped onion, garlic, carrot and fennel on medium heat for 5-6 minutes. Add stock and bring to the boil; reduce heat and simmer for 10 minutes.

Add zucchini and green beans, bring back to the boil and cook for another 10 minutes. Next, add navy beans and tomatoes and simmer for a further five minutes.

While the soup is cooking, prepare the *pistou*. In a small blender, combine garlic, basil leaves, olive oil, salt and pepper and pulse until smooth.

Stir *pistou* sauce gently into the hot soup and combine carefully. Ladle into soup bowls and garnish with basil leaves. Serve hot or at room temperature.

2 tbsp olive oil

1 onion, chopped

2 cloves garlic, finely chopped

2 carrots, peeled and finely diced

1 fennel bulb, finely diced

2 medium zucchini, cut into cubes

11oz/300g green beans, topped, tailed and coarsely chopped

11oz/300g navy beans, precooked or from a jar

15oz/400g (approx. 4 medium) tomatoes, skinned, seeded and cubed, or15oz/400g tomatoes in a jar

2 pints/1l vegetable or chicken stock

Pistou

3 cloves garlic, crushed

5-6 tbsp chopped basil (saving 6 leaves for garnish)

1 fl oz/2-3 tbsp/30 ml olive oil

salt & freshly ground black pepper

Cool minty cucumber soup

2 tbsp almond slivers

3 tbsp mint leaves

7oz/scant cup/200g plain
yogurt

1 large cucumber, cubed

zest and juice of ½ lemon

3 tbsp olive oil

1oz/4 tbsp/30g ground
almonds

1 clove garlic, crushed

1 small apple, peeled,
cored and cubed

salt & freshly ground
black pepper

pinch red pepper flakes or
paprika powder

On a hot summer's day, the mere thought of this pale-green, minty concoction will send cool waves through you. What's more, you won't work up a sweat as it is ready in a matter of minutes and there is next-to-no cooking involved! Serves 4.

In a dry skillet and on low heat, lightly toast almond slivers for 1-2 minutes until barely golden. Transfer to a plate to cool.

Pick the mint leaves off the stalks, set a few aside for garnish and place the rest in a blender along with yogurt, cucumber, lemon juice and zest, olive oil, almonds, crushed garlic and apple. Blend until smooth and light green. Adjust seasoning to taste. Chill for at least 1 hour; this allows the flavors to deepen.

Serve in individual bowls or glasses decorated with mint leaves. Sprinkle lightly with pepper flakes or paprika powder and toasted almond slivers. For extra cooling effect, add 1-2 ice cubes per glass.

Variation
Replace the mint with 1-2 tbsp chopped dill and garnish the soup with a teaspoonful of salmon roe for a Scandinavian touch.

Chilled garlic and almond soup

This refreshing garlicky soup from southern Spain, *sopa de ajo blanco*, is a wonderful antidote to scorching summer heat: nourishing and soothing, it does not weigh you down despite its high-calorie ingredients. The traditional recipe calls for soaked bread but I find it just as delicious, and more refreshing, without. Make sure you use fresh garlic as you will be eating it raw. Remove any green sprouts from the garlic cloves before crushing these or the soup may get a little too pungent. Serves 4.

Place almonds in a blender, add olive oil, vinegar, salt and squeeze garlic into the blender with a garlic press. Blend at high speed until the mixture is smooth; add cold water and keep blending. If you find the texture too thick, add a little more water. Season to taste with salt and vinegar.

Pour soup into serving bowl and chill for at least 1 hour. To chill it faster, place bowl in a larger basin filled with ice water for 5-10 minutes.

Serve in individual soup bowls or glasses, with an added ice cube for extra coolness and garnished with halved, de-seeded grapes.

7oz/200g blanched whole or slivered almonds

5fl oz/⅔ cup/150ml extra virgin olive oil

2-3 cloves garlic

1 tbsp sherry vinegar

salt

13½ fl oz/1¾ cups/400ml chilled water

12 white grapes, halved and de-seeded, as garnish

Gazpacho with avocado relish

1¾lb/800g fresh, sun-ripened tomatoes, cubed

2 red bell peppers, chopped

1 cucumber, cubed

1 purple onion, chopped

3 tbsp fresh chopped basil

1-2 cloves garlic, crushed

2.5fl oz/¹/₃ cup/75ml extra virgin olive oil

3 tbsp tomato paste

2fl oz/¼ cup/50ml sherry vinegar or red-wine vinegar

salt & freshly ground black pepper

Avocado relish

1 ripe avocado, peeled, pitted and cubed

1 tomato, finely chopped

1 spring onion, chopped

1 tbsp cilantro, chopped

1 tbsp olive oil

1 tbsp lemon juice

salt & freshly ground black pepper

Another refreshing soup from Spain's sun-scorched south. Contrary to the chilled garlic soup, this one is packed with vegetables, making it lighter and brimming with protective plant compounds. These may require more prep time, but since none of it demands much precision – just a bit of coarse chopping and shredding – it's easily done. If you can't get hold of cilantro, you can replace it with basil, parsley or chives, or a combination of these. Serves 4.

Combine tomatoes, peppers, cucumber, onion and basil in a large salad bowl and squeeze the garlic into the vegetables with a garlic press; add olive oil, tomato paste and vinegar and toss to combine.

Tip about half the mixture into a blender and liquidize. Transfer to a serving bowl. Blend the second batch and combine with the first. Season with salt and pepper. Place in the refrigerator for at least 2 hours to allow the flavors to infuse.

Just before serving, prepare relish: combine cubed avocados, spring onion, tomato, cilantro and lemon juice in a bowl, toss lightly and season to taste with salt and pepper. To serve, place an ice cube or two in each serving bowl or glass, ladle soup over these and top with avocado garnish.

Variation
Garnishing gazpacho with hard-boiled, chopped egg boosts the protein content of this dish and makes it suitable for a stand-alone meal.

Eggs

Eggs are a tasty, versatile, inexpensive and easily available source of high-quality protein. They contain the anti-inflammatory compound choline and the antioxidant lutein and have also been found to encourage weight loss and boost eye sight, brain and nervous system function.

Although they all look the same, not all eggs are alike, however; their nutritional quality depends on what the hens that laid them ate. The six hens we keep in our garden eat slugs, snails, worms, the occasional frog, grass seeds and grains including flax seeds. Their eggs taste sweet and buttery and the yolks have a deep orange color.

Eggs from intensively reared hens fed only cereal grains contain nearly 20 times more of the inflammatory omega-6 fatty acids than anti-inflammatory omega-3s (see p. 44-5). Yet, their eggs look just like eggs from chickens that have roamed free and foraged for their own food.

When you buy your eggs, therefore, read labels carefully. Check how the hens were raised, whether they had access to open land under open skies, and what they were fed. Some farmers now feed their hens flax seeds to increase their eggs' omega-3 content; these are marked "omega-3 enriched" on the label. However, this does not necessarily mean they were raised outdoors, nor that they were fed organically, unless specifically stated.

If you have a garden, consider keeping a few hens – they're easy to keep and require no looking after except for occasional coop clean-outs. They can be quite companionable – ours allow us to stroke them! If this seems too extreme, talk to farmers selling their eggs at the market and ask them how their hens are raised and fed. With a bit of luck, you might find someone who keeps hens the "old-fashioned" way.

Always make sure you buy the freshest eggs possible by checking the date stamped on the box. The freshest ones are usually at the very back of the shelf; there can be a difference of a week between the ones in the front and the ones in the back. Before you put the carton in your basket, check that none of the eggs are cracked.

At home, you can test whether an egg is fresh by filling a bowl with water and placing the egg in it; if it sinks, it's fine, if it floats, discard it – it's too old to eat.

Three frittatas

A frittata is an Italian omelet filled with vegetables, pasta or meat and a great way of using up leftovers. Enjoy it hot or cold, for breakfast, lunch and dinner, at picnics or in a lunchbox. All recipes serve 4.

Spinach and goats' cheese frittata

2 tbsp olive oil

1 onion, finely chopped

1 clove garlic, finely chopped

1.1lb/450g fresh or frozen (defrosted) leaf spinach

5 eggs

3½ fl oz/scant ½ cup/ 100ml milk

grated nutmeg

7oz/200g fresh goats' cheese, cubed

2 tbsp toasted pine nuts

salt & freshly ground black pepper

In a heavy cooking pot warm 1 tablespoon olive oil and cook onions and garlic for 4-5 minutes, or until translucent. Add spinach and keep stirring until wilted (about 3 minutes). Tip spinach-onion mix into a strainer and squeeze out excess moisture.

While the spinach is draining, whisk eggs and milk together in a mixing bowl, seasoning with salt, pepper and nutmeg. Add drained spinach to egg mixture and combine. Fold in goats' cheese, taking care not to squash cubes.

Reheat skillet and add 1 tablespoon olive oil. Pour egg mixture into pan and cook for about 10 minutes on medium heat; sprinkle with pine nuts, place pan under grill and cook for another 2-3 minutes until pine nuts are golden.

Leek and salmon frittata

In a skillet on medium heat, warm 2 tablespoons of olive oil and cook leeks and garlic for 8 minutes, stirring regularly. Add a splash of water or white wine and cover with a lid if they brown. Remove from heat and set aside.

In a bowl, beat eggs with lemon zest, dill and mustard, add milk, whisk and season with salt and pepper. Add leeks and salmon and fold in gently.

Wipe frying pan clean with a paper towel, place on medium heat, add the remaining tablespoon olive oil and warm. Reduce heat to low setting, pour egg, leek and fish mixture into the pan and cook for 5-6 minutes while pre-heating the grill to medium. Place skillet under grill and cook for a further 4 minutes until the fish is cooked through and the egg is puffy and golden.

3 tbsp olive oil
4 medium leeks, sliced
1 clove garlic, chopped
5 eggs
3½ fl oz/scant ½ cup/ 100ml milk
grated zest of ¼ lemon
1 tbsp chopped dill weed
1 tbsp grainy mustard
10 oz/300g fresh salmon, cubed
salt & pepper

Mixed vegetable and tofu frittata

In a skillet over medium heat, warm 2 tablespoons olive oil and cook onions and garlic for 4-5 minutes. Add quartered mushrooms and cook for another 5-6 minutes. Transfer to a bowl and set aside.

Return the pan to moderate heat, add another tablespoon of olive oil and cook tofu cubes until golden on all sides – around 10 minutes. Remove from heat and set aside. While tofu is browning, steam broccoli and zucchini for 5 minutes until tender but *al dente*. Remove and set aside.

In a bowl, beat eggs and milk, add parsley and season with salt and pepper. Add onions, mushrooms, broccoli, zucchini and tofu cubes and combine well.

Return the skillet to low heat, add 1 tablespoon olive oil, pour egg, vegetable and tofu mixture into pan and cook for 5 minutes on medium heat; sprinkle with chopped hazelnuts, and grill for 3-4 minutes or until egg is set.

4 tbsp olive oil
1 onion, sliced
2 cloves garlic, chopped
7oz/200g mushrooms
7oz/200g tofu, cubed
1 zucchini, sliced
5-6 broccoli florets
5 eggs
3½ fl oz/scant cup/ 100ml unsweetened almond milk
2 tbsp chopped parsley
2 tbsp chopped hazelnuts
salt & pepper

Cherry tomato *clafoutis*

15oz/400g cherry tomatoes, washed and patted dry

7oz/200g feta cheese, crumbled

2 tbsp corn starch

4 eggs

12fl oz/1½ cups/350ml unsweetened almond or soy milk

large pinch of turmeric (to taste)

2 tbsp chopped chives or basil leaves

salt & freshly ground black pepper

some olive oil for the pie dish

Clafoutis, a classic French dish, is most widely known in its original incarnation as a sweet cherry pie. This savory version makes a quick and easy summer lunch when tomatoes are sweet and aromatic and juicy herbs abound. Tastes great with Warm Puy lentil salad (p. 187) or with a lightly tossed green salad. Serves 4.

Preheat oven to 350°F/180°C.

Oil oven-proof ceramic dish and place cherry tomatoes and crumbled feta cheese in it.

In a bowl, whisk corn starch with milk and eggs. Add half the chopped herbs and turmeric and combine into a smooth, creamy batter. Season with salt and pepper.

Pour egg mixture gently over tomatoes and feta cheese and slide the pie dish into the oven. Bake for approximately 30 minutes. The *clafoutis* is ready when the custard has risen and is a golden color.

Remove from the oven, sprinkle with remaining herbs and serve immediately.

Green soufflé

While soufflés don't appreciate sudden changes in temperature, they are otherwise undemanding creatures. You can prepare most of this in advance, leaving only a few minutes of egg-white-whipping and baking for the end. To speed things up, bake and serve these in individual ramekins (careful: hot!). Serves 4.

Preheat oven with a baking tray at its center to 425°F/220°C. Grease soufflé dish or ramekins up to the rim and dust with finely ground pecorino or Parmesan cheese.

In a medium pot, heat 1 tablespoon olive oil and cook chopped onions and garlic until translucent, about 4-5 minutes. Add spinach, broccoli and 4-5 tablespoons water and cook, covered, until the broccoli is *al dente* (5-6 minutes). Tip into a food processor fitted with an S-shaped blade and puree until smooth.

Rinse the pot, combine in it cold milk, flour and 4 tablespoons olive oil and gently heat, stirring constantly to prevent lumps as the mixture thickens. Remove from heat, cool for 5 minutes, add nutmeg and egg yolks, vegetable puree and half the goats' cheese. Season with salt and pepper.

Beat egg whites in a clean, dry bowl with an electric whisk until they are firm, adding a pinch of salt halfway through. Beat one tablespoon of egg white into the vegetable mixture to slacken it, then fold in the remaining egg whites with a metal spoon. Do not beat – just fold in gently.

Pour soufflé mixture into the prepared dish, sprinkle with the remaining cheese and place on baking tray in the preheated oven, lowering thermostat to 375°F/190°C immediately. Bake until set and golden, about 30 minutes for a large dish or 15-20 minutes for ramekins.

olive oil and 2-3 tbsp grated pecorino or Parmesan to line soufflé dish

5 tbsp olive oil

1 small onion, finely chopped

2 cloves garlic, finely chopped

7oz/200g leaf spinach, thoroughly washed and coarsely chopped

9oz/250g broccoli, coarsely chopped

1 heaped tbsp whole grain wheat or spelt flour

5fl oz/⅔ cup/150ml unsweetened almond or soy milk

grated nutmeg

4 egg yolks

2½ oz/70g feta cheese (or soft goat's cheese)

5 egg whites

Onion *clafoutis*

2 tbsp olive oil

1.1lb/500g (approx. 3 large) red onions, halved and thinly sliced

½ tsp thyme

1 heaped tbsp corn starch

1 tsp turmeric

3 large or 4 small eggs

5fl oz/⅔ cup/150ml unsweetened almond or soy milk

salt & freshly ground black pepper

The French are masters at the art of *gratins*: vegetables or fruit covered with egg custard or cheese, baked golden in the oven and served straight out of attractive ceramic dishes. Their ease of preparation (everything goes into the same dish, which is the only one you'll have to wash up!) makes them a boon for the busy cook, and they're a great way of using up leftovers. Here, red onions – richer in protective plant chemicals than their yellow cousins – offer striking visual appeal. Serves 4.

Preheat oven to 350°F/180°C. Grease an oven-proof ceramic dish.

Heat olive oil in a pan on low heat and slowly stew onions and thyme without letting them color or turn crisp; if they get too dry, add a little water. Stir gently every now and then to avoid sticking, but be careful not to mash the onions with overly enthusiastic stirring. Cook for about 20 minutes until soft and sweet.

In a mixing bowl, beat corn starch, turmeric and eggs and slowly add milk, whisking steadily until you obtain a smooth batter. When the onions are soft, cool for 5 minutes and then stir into the batter. Season with salt and pepper.

Pour into oven-proof dish and bake in preheated oven for 20-25 minutes or until puffed and golden. Serve immediately accompanied by a mixed salad or green vegetable.

Basque *piperade*

This late-summer delicacy from the French Basque country is a wonderful all-rounder: perfect as a light lunch, delicious for dinner with crisply steamed green beans or lightly dressed lettuce leaves, and even on a slice of grilled wholegrain toast for breakfast the next day. It takes at most 30 minutes to make, so it can be rustled up quickly at the end of a long day! Serves 4.

In a large, heavy-bottomed pan, warm the olive oil and gently cook onions and garlic until they are translucent (4-5 minutes). Add peppers, tomatoes, herbs and pepper flakes and continue cooking for about 15 minutes, stirring occasionally. Season to taste with salt and pepper. If the tomatoes are acidic, a smidgen of honey will soften their flavor.

While the vegetables are cooking, crack the eggs into a small mixing bowl and beat lightly with a fork. When the vegetables are quite soft, gently stir the eggs into the peppers, continue cooking and stirring for a minute and then remove from the heat; this way the eggs will set but won't get too firm. Sprinkle with chopped parsley and serve immediately.

Variation

If you don't like mixing the eggs into the vegetables, spread the vegetables evenly across the pan and with a large spoon, press four hollows into them into which you crack the eggs. Place the pan in an oven preheated to 350°F/180°C for 5-6 minutes until the egg whites are set but the yolks remain runny. If desired, sprinkle eggs with grated ewes' milk cheese before popping the pan into the oven for a delicious melted effect.

---

2 large tbsp olive oil

1 large or 2 small onions, peeled, quartered and sliced

2 cloves garlic, finely chopped

3 bell peppers (I like to use 1 green, 1 red and 1 yellow, but choose any colors you like), halved, de-seeded and sliced about ¼ inch/5mm wide

4-5 large, ripe tomatoes (or 15oz/400 g tomatoes out of a jar), chopped

½ tsp thyme, 1 bay leaf

large pinch of Piment d'Espelette or mild red pepper flakes

1 tsp acacia honey (optional)

4 eggs

1 tbsp chopped parsley

salt & freshly ground black pepper

Porcini omelet

3-4 eggs

2 tbsp olive oil

salt & freshly ground black pepper

½ quantity Mushrooms Bordelaise (p. 214)

If you can't get hold of fresh porcini mushrooms (their season is quite short), you can use pretty much any firm mushroom, such as shiitake, oyster, chestnut or even white button mushrooms; the darker, wilder varieties offer more flavor and cancer-fighting nutrients than the lighter ones. A tasty compromise would be standard button mushrooms complemented with 3 or 4 rehydrated, chopped dried porcini, which you should be able to find year round in well-stocked supermarkets or health-food shops. Frozen mushrooms work well too. Serves 2.

First, prepare mushroom filling following the recipe for Mushrooms *Bordelaise* (p. 214), halving the quantity (for 2 persons). Keep these warm while you prepare the omelet.

Break eggs into a mixing bowl, add 1 tbsp water per egg, season lightly with salt and pepper, and whisk with a fork until loosely mixed.

In a skillet on medium heat, warm olive oil and pour in the beaten eggs. With a spatula, gently lift up the edges of the omelet and tilt and rotate the pan to allow uncooked egg to flow underneath.

While the top is still moist and creamy, cover one half of the omelet with the mushrooms. Slip the spatula under the unfilled side, flip it over the mushrooms, thus folding the omelet in half, and slide onto a warmed serving dish.

Sardine omelet

Bored with canned sardines on toast? Here's a tasty and speedy way of enjoying this omega-3 rich delicacy. This is delicious as a weekend breakfast served with rye toast or as a light lunch with mixed salad or steamed vegetables.
I like green peppers here, but you can also use red or yellow peppers, asparagus, fresh firm tomatoes, zucchini or any other tasty vegetable that strikes your fancy. Serves 2.

Heat 1 tablespoon olive oil in a medium-sized skillet and gently cook onion and garlic for 2 minutes, then add pepper. Continue cooking until pepper has softened slightly (4-5 minutes). Remove from heat and tip vegetables into a bowl; set aside.

Warm a second tablespoon of oil in the same pan and cook the sardines on both sides. Remove to a plate and break up coarsely with a fork. Wipe skillet with a paper towel.

In another bowl, whisk eggs, chopped parsley, salt and pepper and a pinch of turmeric. Heat the remaining tablespoon of olive oil in the pan and pour in the beaten egg. Spread fish, onion and pepper mix on top and leave to cook on a low heat until the omelet is almost set.

Slide onto a preheated serving plate, folding the omelet in half as you do so.

3 tbsp olive oil

2 spring onions (or half a regular onion), coarsely chopped

1 clove garlic, finely chopped

1 green pepper, deseeded and cubed

7oz/200g fresh sardine fillets or 2 BPA-free cans whole sardines in olive oil, drained

3-4 eggs

1 tbsp chopped parsley

pinch of turmeric

salt & freshly ground black pepper

Spanish sweet-potato omelet

5 tbsp olive oil

1 large onion, coarsely chopped

4-5 cloves garlic, finely chopped

2 medium sweet potatoes, peeled and cut into cubes of approx. roughly ½ inch by ½ inch (1 x 1 cm)

4 eggs

½ tsp rosemary, finely chopped

salt and pepper

Tortilla de patatas (potato omelet) is a Spanish tapa classic. To offset the potatoes' sweetness, I've flavored this tortilla with rosemary, onions and plenty of garlic. Feel free to add other ingredients, such as cubes of red or green peppers, zucchini, peas, olives or finely chopped chilies. For extra seasoning and color, you can add paprika powder and turmeric. Serves 4 as *hors d'oeuvre* or more for a snack.

In a medium skillet, warm 4 tablespoons olive oil and add onion, garlic and potatoes; sprinkle with salt and cover.

Cook slowly on low to medium heat, turning the vegetables every 5 minutes with a spatula to cook them evenly. If the onions start turning crispy, add 2-3 tablespoons of water. The potatoes should take about 15-20 minutes to soften (the smaller the cubes, the faster they will cook through).

Meanwhile, break eggs into a mixing bowl and beat with a fork. Season with salt and pepper, add rosemary. When the vegetables are *al dente*, remove from heat, cool for 5 minutes, tip into the egg mixture and gently combine.

Add 1 tablespoon olive oil to the skillet and place back on the heat; pour contents of the bowl into the skillet, spread evenly and turn heat to lowest setting. Cook gently for 8-10 minutes until the underside of the omelet is golden-brown; the surface may still be quite wobbly.

Slide the omelet onto a large, flat plate, place skillet upside-down over the plate and flip both over so that the cooked side of the omelet is now facing upwards in the pan. Return pan to heat and cook for another 2 minutes until the egg is set, and slide onto serving plate. Cool until lukewarm; cut into wedges or cubes to serve.

Fish

Since the Mediterranean basin is by definition a maritime region, its inhabitants have traditionally eaten a diet rich in fish and seafood.

Thanks to the influx of cold water from the Atlantic Ocean through the Straits of Gibraltar, the Mediterranean is, among others, home to fatty cold-water fish such as anchovies, sardines, sea bass, mackerel, sea bream and tuna.

Alas, the sea is suffering from the effects of pollution from industry, shipping and intensive tourism. Overfishing, too, is a problem; some of the most important fisheries in the Mediterranean, such as blue fin and albacore tuna, hake, marlin, swordfish, red mullet and sea bream, are threatened. This is why it's wise to vary the types of fish you eat, and to choose smaller, less polluted and less threatened varieties such as sardines.

As we noted earlier, fish is a very useful part of an anti-cancer diet. Most importantly, fatty fish contains beneficial oils rich in omega-3 fatty acids. Oily fish is also an excellent source of important anti-cancer vitamins and minerals – vitamin D, selenium and iodine – that are not easily found in other foods. Moreover, it offers a healthy alternative to meat by providing high-quality protein that our bodies need to stay healthy and build and repair tissue.

Thus, we should aim to eat fish regularly - ideally, two to three times a week. Fresh fish tastes best, but frozen (plain, raw) fish is a good choice too, and more convenient for people who do not have the time to shop for fresh fish several times a week.

One reason why many of us don't cook fish at home is that we do not know how to prepare it. Granted, fish is more delicate than meat, making it less suited to certain preparations. Over the next few pages, however, you will discover many quick and easy ways of preparing fish: simmered in an aromatic broth, oven-roasted, grilled, braised, topped with crunchy breadcrumbs or steamed in a *papillotte* parcel.

Provençal salmon parcels

4 tomatoes, fresh or from a jar, coarsely chopped

2 spring onions, thinly sliced

1 clove garlic, crushed

2 tbsp olive oil

½ tsp herbes de Provence

4 salmon steaks

4 heaped tsp olive tapenade (p. 122)

2 lemons slices, cut in half

4 generous pinches thyme

salt & freshly ground black pepper

four squares each of baking parchment and aluminum foil, roughly 12 by 12 inches (30 by 30 cm) in size

If you're unsure how to cook fish, this dish is a great place to start. All you need are fresh salmon fillets, some green-olive tapenade (shop-bought, or home-made using the recipe on p. 122, replacing black with green olives), tomatoes and spring onions. This also tastes great cold, so why not make a double batch and take leftovers to work the next day? Serves 4.

Preheat oven to 350°F/180°C.

In a small mixing bowl, combine chopped tomatoes, spring onions or garlic, olive oil, *herbes de Provence*, salt and pepper and stir until mixed.

Lay out 4 squares of aluminum foil and place 4 squares of baking parchment on top of these. Spoon tomato mix onto each square – about 2 tablespoons per parcel – and place salmon steaks on top. Spread each steak with 1-2 teaspoons of *tapenade*, place half a lemon slice on top and sprinkle with thyme.

Now fold over the edges of the parchment and foil squares and scrunch up the edges tightly. The parcels should be well sealed so that no steam can escape during cooking, keeping the fish nice and moist. Place parcels on baking tray and slide into preheated oven. Bake for 15-20 minutes, depending on the size of the salmon fillets. When serving, gently undo foil and slide contents of the parcels onto dining plates.

Variations
- Braised fennel and onions (p. 211) make a delicious base.
- Ratatouille (p. 222) also works well as a base.

Chermoula-stuffed sardines

Chermoula, the fragrant north African herb-and-spice paste on p. 228, helps to mask the oily flavor of fresh sardines, resulting in a fresh and aromatic fish dish. A little advance planning is required, but the preparation itself is as simple as can be. Serves 4.

To stuff the sardine fillets: take a fillet and place it skin side down. Spread the fillet with about one teaspoon of *chermoula*. Take a second fillet, slather it with *chermoula* too and sandwich the two together, skin sides facing out. Cover and refrigerate for at least one hour, preferably two to three.

Place flour on a plate, season with salt and pepper and dredge the fish in it on both sides; shake off excess flour and set aside.

Meanwhile, cover the bottom of a large skillet with olive oil and warm over medium heat. Cook the sardine "sandwiches" 3-4 minutes on each side, or until golden. Drain on paper towels before transferring to a warmed serving plate.

Serve with lemon wedges and a crisp mixed salad or steamed greens.

1.3lb/600g fresh sardine fillets (scaled, rinsed and patted dry with paper towels)

3-4 tbsp whole wheat or spelt flour, or corn flour

salt & freshly ground black pepper

olive oil

1 portion Chermoula (p. 228)

Express Bouillabaisse

4 tbsp olive oil

1 onion, finely chopped

1 clove garlic, finely chopped

1 leek, finely sliced (white and light-green sections only)

1 rib celery, finely chopped

1 bulb fennel, quartered, cored and finely sliced; reserve fronds for garnish

1l water

1 fish or vegetable bouillon cube

4fl oz/½ cup/120ml white wine

4 fresh tomatoes, chopped (or 15oz/400g tomatoes from a jar)

½ tsp thyme

2 bay leaves

1 tsp fennel seeds, generous pinch of saffron

2 inches/5cm thinly pared orange peel (organic)

1 salmon fillet (approx. 9oz/250g)

8 red mullet fillets (scaled)

1.1lb/500g of firm white fish fillets (e.g. haddock, sea bass)

There are as many Mediterranean fish stew recipes as there are fish in the sea, but the most famous is probably Bouillabaisse from Marseille. This is a quick-and-easy version of that delicious but time-consuming traditional dish. In contrast to the delicately flavored soup, *rouille*, a garlic-and-olive-oil mayonnaise traditionally served on crusty bread croutons alongside Bouillabaisse, adds a welcome kick. You can use any firm-fleshed varieties of ocean fish your fishmonger might recommend, but try to include red mullet, which adds a beautiful orange hue, a rich iodine flavor and omega-3 fats. Serves 4-6.

In a large, heavy-bottomed pot, heat olive oil on medium heat and gently cook the chopped onion and garlic until translucent (4-5 minutes). Add leeks, celery and fennel and cook until these begin to soften. Add water and crumbled bouillon cube, white wine, tomatoes, herbs, spices and orange peel. Bring to the boil, then simmer on low heat until all the vegetables are tender – about 15 minutes. (This can be prepared in advance.)

About 10 minutes before you plan to eat, gently re-heat soup base. Carefully lay the fish portions into the liquid, barely submerging them. Do not stir as the pieces of fish should retain their shape. Simmer on low heat until the fish loses its transparency, but be careful not to overcook (about 5 minutes).

Season to taste with salt and pepper, sprinkle with chopped parsley and chopped fennel greens.

Rouille

While the soup is simmering, separate egg yolk and white and place yolk in a small mixing bowl. (Store the white in a well-sealed container in the refrigerator.)

Mix yolk with crushed garlic, a pinch of salt and a generous squeeze of lemon juice. Using an electric whisk, beat egg yolk and garlic and then very slowly add oil to the egg mixture: at first in small drops, mixing well, then growing to a thin trickle as the mayonnaise comes together. Whisk steadily while the mixture thickens.

When all the oil has been amalgamated, add more lemon juice and salt and pepper to taste.

Toast thin slices of sourdough bread, spread with *rouille* and serve with the soup. Some like to eat the toast on the side, others prefer to place it afloat on their soup to soak up its saffrony flavors.

As rouille *is made with raw egg yolk, it should not be eaten by pregnant women or people with weakened immune systems. In its place, you can use 3.5oz/100g of commercial olive-oil mayonnaise to which you add 1-2 cloves of crushed garlic and a pinch of saffron.*

2 tbsp chopped parsley

squeeze of lemon juice

salt & freshly ground black pepper

Rouille and croutons

1 egg yolk (organic)

1 clove garlic, finely crushed

lemon juice

3.5fl oz/scant ½ cup/100ml olive oil

1 slice of wholegrain sourdough bread per person

salt & freshly ground black pepper

Fish *plaki*

3 tbsp olive oil

2 onions, halved and thinly sliced

2 cloves garlic, chopped

1 rib celery, finely cubed

2 carrots, finely cubed

2.5fl oz/⅓ cup/75ml water or vegetable stock

2.5fl oz/⅓ cup/75ml white wine

2 large tomatoes, chopped (or ½ 15 oz/400g jar of tomatoes)

pinch of oregano

12 coarsely chopped black olives

1.3lb/600 g firm white fish cut into steaks or fillets

3 thin slices untreated lemon

2 tbsp chopped parsley

salt & freshly ground black pepper

One of the most popular ways of preparing fish in Greece, this dish is eaten hot in winter and lukewarm or cold as a refreshing summer meal. Leaving it to sit for a few hours after cooking allows the flavors to infuse and deepen. Serves 4.

Preheat oven to 350°F/180°C.

In a medium pot soften the onions in the olive oil for 5 minutes. Add garlic, celery, carrots, water, wine, salt and pepper. Cover and simmer for 10 minutes until the carrots are *al dente*, then add tomatoes, olives and oregano and cook for another 5 minutes, covered.

Lay fish steaks or fillets in a lightly oiled ovenproof dish, pour the sauce over it, lay lemon slices on top and cover with foil. Slide into oven and cook for 30 minutes or until the fish flakes easily when prodded with a sharp kitchen knife.

Remove from oven, leave to cool for 5 minutes (if eating hot), sprinkle with parsley and serve. Alternatively, cool and serve at room temperature.

Variation

For a complete meal, I sometimes place the fish on a layer of cooked Garlicky spinach (p. 220) and bake the whole lot together.

Mediterranean baked fish

Many people are afraid to cook fish because it is so delicate in texture and flavor and they're afraid of "getting it wrong." In fact, the less you do to fish, the better it tastes and the less scope there is for mistakes. This typically Mediterranean recipe for gently roasted sea bream is a case in point: cooking doesn't really get any simpler than this. The most important thing here is top-quality, fresh fish. You can spot it by its bright, shiny eyes and absence of a "fishy" smell. Serves 4.

Preheat oven to 350°F/180°C.

Rinse fish under cold running water and pat dry. Rub with olive oil and lightly salt and pepper, inside and out. With a sharp knife, slice two deep slashes sideways into the thickest part of each fish and slide half a bay leaf and half a lemon slice into each flap. Set aside.

In a skillet, warm 1 tablespoon olive oil and cook shallots and garlic on medium heat until translucent. Add tomatoes and herbs, cook for another 10 minutes and season with salt and pepper. Transfer to an ovenproof dish and spread out evenly.

Place fish on top of the onions and tomatoes, drizzle with wine and slide the dish into the hot oven. Bake for approximately 20-25 minutes. To test for doneness, carefully probe the thickest part of the flesh with the tip of a sharp kitchen knife; it should be opaque all the way through.

When the fish is done, remove from the oven, season lightly with salt and pepper, drizzle with the remaining olive oil and serve immediately.

---

2 large or 4 small sea bream, scaled and gutted

3-4 tbsp olive oil

4 thin lemon slices (untreated), each slice cut in half

4 large bay leaves cut in half with scissors

2 shallots, finely sliced

2 cloves garlic, finely chopped

15oz/400g tomatoes, cubed

2 tbsp fresh herbs (parsley, thyme, oregano, dill)

2fl oz/60ml white wine

salt & freshly ground black pepper

Garlic-crusted baked cod

4 tbsp olive oil

4 cloves garlic, chopped

15oz/400 g tomatoes, coarsely chopped (fresh or from a jar)

pinch of mixed herbs (bay leaf, rosemary, oregano)

1.5lb/700g cod or other firm-fleshed fish

2 tbsp flour

salt & freshly ground black pepper

Garlic crust

1 egg, yolk and egg white placed in two separate bowls

2 cloves garlic, crushed

1 pinch paprika powder

4fl oz/½ cup/120ml olive oil

squeeze of lemon juice

salt & freshly ground black pepper

This recipe is inspired by the delicious Catalan dish *bacalao a la muselina de ajo*, though here I have replaced the traditional salted cod with fresh cod. Serve the fish on a light tomato sauce, or perhaps on a bed of Garlicky spinach (p. 220). Serves 4.

Start with the tomato sauce: put 2 tablespoons olive oil into a medium sized pot and cook the chopped garlic for 30-40 seconds until soft but not golden. Add tomatoes and herbs and cook for 15-20 minutes. Season with salt and pepper and transfer to an ovenproof ceramic dish.

Drain the fish, pat dry and lightly toss in flour. Pour remaining olive oil into a skillet and cook fish on low heat for 3-4 minutes on each side, depending on the fish's thickness. Place atop the tomato sauce in the ceramic dish, cover with foil and keep warm. Preheat grill on medium setting.

Prepare garlic crust: place egg yolk, crushed garlic, pepper, salt and paprika in a small bowl. Using an electric whisk, beat these until combined and then add oil to the egg mixture: at first in small drops, mixing well, then growing to a thin trickle as the mayonnaise comes together. Whisk steadily while the mixture thickens. When all the oil has been amalgamated, add lemon juice, salt and pepper to taste.

Wash and dry beaters and whisk the egg whites until firm. Fold the egg whites into the mayonnaise to obtain a smooth, fluffy mousse. Spread an even layer of this garlicky mousse over the fish and grill until golden (approximately 2-3 minutes). Serve immediately.

Sardine crumble

Here you can enjoy the contrast of meltingly soft sardines and crunchy topping. It's easy, inexpensive, packed with anti-cancer ingredients (omega-3 fats, garlic, olive oil, spices and lemon zest) and has a distinctly Mediterranean flavor. Accompanied by a tomato salad with a tangy dressing or a crisp green vegetable, this works well as a simple dinner dish. Serves 4 as a main course.

Preheat oven to 350°F/180°C.

Warm 2 tablespoons olive oil in a skillet on medium heat and cook onion 4-5 minutes until translucent. Add sardines and cook for 2-3 minutes, trying to keep the fish in relatively large chunks. Season with salt, pepper and herbs and spoon equal amounts into 4 ramekins. Drizzle with lemon juice and set aside.

In a small mixing bowl, combine bread crumbs, sesame seeds, garlic, parsley, paprika powder, lemon zest, olive oil, pepper and salt and mix well to obtain a lightly oiled (but not sticky) crumble mix.

Now spoon breadcrumb mix over the sardines, press down lightly, place on a baking tray and slide into the oven. Bake for 15 minutes or until the topping is golden and crispy. Serve with a wedge of lemon.

Variation

For a gluten-free alternative, you can replace the breadcrumbs with plain, low-salt tortilla chips ground up in a food processor to resemble coarse breadcrumbs. Then continue as above.

---

3 tbsp olive oil

1 onion, finely chopped

15oz/400g fresh sardine fillets, or whole sardines in a jar or BPA-free tin, packed in olive oil, drained

squeeze of lemon juice

3.5oz/100g whole grain breadcrumbs

2 tbsp raw sesame seeds

2 cloves garlic, crushed

1 tbsp parsley, finely chopped

½ tsp paprika powder

pinch finely grated lemon zest (untreated)

pinch of herbes de Provence

salt & freshly ground black pepper

Grilled trout with almond-sesame crunch

4 small whole trout, gutted, cleaned and patted dry

3 tbsp olive oil plus more for dish

1 clove garlic, finely chopped

3.5oz/heaped ½ cup/100g whole, skinned almonds, coarsely chopped

2oz/¹⁄₃ cup/50g whole sesame seeds

1 tbsp finely chopped parsley

salt & freshly ground black pepper

4 lemon wedges as garnish

This dish requires only a handful of ingredients, but these need to be of maximum freshness and quality: squeaky-fresh fish (you can recognize it by its clear, shiny eyes and fresh, non-fishy smell); fresh nuts and seeds and top-quality olive oil. Once you've got these assembled, the rest won't take more than 20 minutes to throw together. Serves 4.

Lightly salt the trout's abdominal cavity. Score skin on both sides a few times. Place in an ovenproof dish rubbed with olive oil and a sprinkling of salt and pepper.

Slide under a hot grill for 5-6 minutes, depending on thickness. Turn and grill another 5-6 minutes. The fish is ready when the skin begins to crisp up and the flesh flakes easily when probed with the tip of a sharp knife.

While the fish is under the grill, warm olive oil in a skillet on medium heat and cook garlic for 30 seconds. Add almonds and stir with a wooden spoon for a minute; then add sesame seeds, stirring for another 1-2 minutes until almonds and seeds are lightly golden and crunchy. Season with salt and pepper and remove from heat.

When the fish is ready, remove from grill, drizzle with a squeeze of lemon juice, and scatter with parsley and with the garlic-almond-sesame mix. Garnish with lemon wedges and serve immediately.

Mackerel with mustard

Mackerel is shamefully underrated: it is rich in omega-3 fatty acids, an excellent source of protein, is generally caught in less-polluted ocean waters and is not threatened with extinction. However, many people find mackerel challenging because of its strong taste, courtesy of said high fat content. Two things can help: buying only the very freshest mackerel (it should ideally smell of "ocean" rather than of "fish") and matching it with other gutsy flavors that can stand up to the fish's assertive taste. I like to combine it with mustard, white wine and onions, which results in an aromatic dish that is quick and easy to prepare and tastes good warm or cold. Serves 4.

Preheat oven to 400°F/200°C.

In a skillet, cook onion and garlic in olive oil with the bay leaf and thyme and a pinch of salt until the onions are translucent (4-5 minutes); transfer to an ovenproof ceramic dish. Lay mackerel fillets on top, pour white wine and water over the fish and season lightly with salt and pepper. Place in the oven and bake uncovered for 15 minutes.

When the fish is cooked-through, remove from the oven and carefully strain the cooking juices into a small pot, leaving the fish and onions in the baking dish. Cover the dish with foil to keep fish warm.

Bring fish juices to the boil and reduce by half. Add mustards, lemon juice, turmeric and Cashew cream, bring to the boil again and stir until thickened (add water if it's too thick). Pour sauce over mackerel fillets in the baking dish, sprinkle with parsley and serve immediately.

---

1 tbsp olive oil

1 large onion, quartered and thinly sliced

1 clove garlic, finely chopped

1 bay leaf

¼ tsp thyme

1.5lb/650 g fresh mackerel fillets

7fl oz/1 scant cup/200ml white wine

3.5fl oz/scant ½ cup/100ml water

1 tbsp Dijon other any other sharp mustard

1 tbsp traditional wholegrain mustard

1-2 tbsp lemon juice (to taste)

pinch of turmeric

3.5fl oz/scant ½ cup/100ml Cashew cream (p. 231)

1 tbsp chopped parsley

salt & freshly ground black pepper

Pesto-baked salmon

2 tbsp olive oil

4 spring onions, sliced

2 cloves garlic, finely chopped

15oz/400g cherry tomatoes

4 salmon fillets

4 tbsp basil pesto, home-made (p. 229) or shop-bought

salt & freshly ground black pepper

Fragrant baked tomatoes and moist salmon under a herby crust make this a perennial favorite in my home. This is quick, simple and works well all year round. Serves 4.

Preheat oven to 350°F/180°C.

In a skillet, cook spring onions and garlic in olive oil for 3-4 minutes, add whole cherry tomatoes and cook another 3 minutes. Season lightly with salt and pepper and transfer to an ovenproof ceramic dish.

Nestle salmon fillets among the tomatoes and, using a teaspoon, spread the tops of the fish with pesto until they are well covered – about 1 tbsp per fillet. Place in a preheated oven and bake for 15-20 minutes. Test for doneness with a kitchen knife – the thinner parts of the fillet should flake easily.

While the salmon is baking, you can prepare a vegetable side dish; this tastes very good with Garlicky spinach (p. 220) or Pumpkin mash (see p. 221).

Marinated sardines

This Spanish classic, *sardinas en escabeche,* is a simple and tasty way to enjoy these omega-3 rich little fish. The highly aromatic marinade cuts through the oily taste of the fish and keeps the sardines fresh in the refrigerator for several days. Serves 4.

Place the flour in a deep plate and dredge sardine fillets in it, shaking off excess flour.

In a skillet on medium heat, heat 3 tablespoons of olive oil, cook half the sardine fillets for 1 minute on each side and transfer to a shallow dish. If necessary, add another tablespoon of olive oil to cook remaining fish.

Now cook onion, garlic, thyme and bay leaf in the same pan. When the onions are soft, add lemon or orange peel, pepper flakes, salt, pepper and vinegar and bring to the boil; reduce heat, cover and simmer for 10-12 minutes.

Remove from heat, add lemon juice and remaining olive oil and pour the warm marinade over the sardines in the dish. Just before serving, sprinkle with chopped parsley.

This dish can be eaten straight away but also tastes good cold, especially after marinating, covered, in the refrigerator for 12 hours or more.

3.5oz/⅔ cup/100g whole wheat, spelt or corn flour

1.3lb/600g fresh sardine fillets (about 18 fish), cleaned, scaled and patted dry with paper towels

2fl oz/¼ cup/60ml olive oil

1 medium red onion, thinly sliced

4 cloves garlic, thinly sliced

½ tsp thyme

1 bay leaf

1 strip untreated orange or lemon peel

pinch of red pepper flakes

1.7fl oz/scant ¼ cup/50ml red-wine vinegar

juice of ½ lemon

2 tbsp coarsely chopped parsley

½ tsp salt, freshly ground black pepper

Fish in a creamy parsley sauce

1 tbsp soft butter

1 finely chopped shallot

1 bay leaf

¼ tsp thyme

1 strip of lemon peel
(about 2 inches/5cm)

4 firm-fleshed fish fillets,
each about 5.5oz/160g

7fl oz/scant 1 cup/200ml
vegetable or fish stock

3.5fl oz/scant ½ cup/100
ml dry white wine

3-4 tbsp finely chopped
parsley

3.5fl oz/scant ½ cup/100
ml Cashew cream (p. 231)

salt & freshly ground
black pepper

squeeze of lemon juice

Lightly poached fish in a herby cream sauce is a French classic. Here I've replaced dairy cream with Cashew cream, which tastes just as comforting but is dairy-free. Any filleted white fish will do, and salmon works well, too. You can use a wide variety of herbs, such as parsley (the easiest to get hold of), dill (a classic fish herb that goes particularly well with salmon) or sorrel (which adds a lightly acidic note). Serves 4.

Preheat oven to 425°F/220°C.

Lightly butter an ovenproof dish, place in it shallots, bay leaf, thyme and lemon peel and lay fish on top. Pour stock and wine over these and bake in preheated oven for 10 minutes or until the fish flakes easily. While the fish is baking, chop the parsley.

One the fish is done, turn off the oven, remove dish and carefully pour the cooking juices into a pan, holding the fish down with a spatula to prevent it sliding out. Return the fish in its dish to the still-warm oven and cover with a piece of foil to prevent drying.

Bring the fish juices to the boil and reduce by half. Add Cashew cream and chopped parsley, stir well and bring back to bubble until the sauce thickens. If it is too thick, add some more water. Season with salt, pepper and lemon juice and pour over the fish in the oven dish; serve immediately.

Serve with colorful vegetables, such as Ruby melt (p. 218), Brussels sprouts (pp. 212-213) or Broccoli-cauliflower medley (p. 215). A vegetable mash – like Pumpkin mash (p. 221) – lends itself to mopping up the sauce.

Poultry and rabbit

Chicken, turkey and rabbit meat, while not anti-cancer foods *per se*, are nevertheless a useful part of an anti-cancer diet. They provide high-quality protein and are easy for most people to digest.

As with all animal foods, it is important to know how the chicken, turkey or rabbit you are eating was raised: cooped-up in crowded, airless battery-farms and kept alive with the help of antibiotics, or with free access to outdoor space and fed natural foods appropriate for its species?

The best way to obtain high-quality meat is to buy it straight from the producer. This meat may cost more than cheap cuts sold in supermarkets, but it will probably be less expensive than meat sold in specialist health-food shops, and fresher, too. Small, traditional butchers who often know the producers of the meat they sell can generally be relied upon to sell high-quality products as well.

I am wary of inexpensive supermarket meat which may come from animals reared on cheap, omega-6-rich feed in cramped conditions; when buying meat at a supermarket, read the label carefully to find out how the animal was fed and reared.

Meat should be as fresh as possible and prepared immediately. For the purposes of cost savings and efficiency, you can purchase larger quantities of meat (for instance, when you buy straight from the farm) and freeze it for later use; freeze immediately to maintain freshness.

As discussed earlier, the healthiest and tastiest way of preparing meat is to cook it gently at moderate temperatures, ideally braising or stewing it in some sort of sauce or broth. Slow cookers are ideally suited to these types of dishes.

Vegetarians may wish to skip this chapter. However, in many of the recipes meat can be replaced by tofu, so it may be worth your while to flick through them to see if any of them sound appetizing.

Chicken and red wine stew

1 chicken (approx. 1½ kg), jointed, or 4 chicken thighs, excess fat removed

9fl oz/1 cup/250 ml red wine

10-12 shallots, whole, or 2 large onions, halved and finely sliced

5 cloves garlic, coarsely chopped

1oz/25g dried porcini or shiitake mushrooms

1 tsp thyme

2-3 bay leaves

4 tbsp olive oil

1 tbsp whole spelt, wheat or corn flour

9fl oz/1 cup/250 ml chicken stock

1.1lb/500g chestnut or button mushrooms

2 tbsp parsley, chopped

untreated fresh grapes for decoration (if available)

salt & freshly ground black pepper

This French classic, *coq au vin*, is crammed with cancer-protective ingredients: onions, garlic, herbs, mushrooms and red wine. It's incredibly easy to make and wonderfully satisfying on a cold, wet winter night. If you marinade the chicken in the wine overnight, the taste is particularly rich; but even rustled up at short notice, it's very tasty. Vegetarians can replace chicken with plain tofu. Serves 4.

Place meat in a sealable container and combine with red wine, shallots or onions, garlic, dried mushrooms, bay leaves and thyme. Seal and marinate overnight, or at least 1-2 hours if you can.

When you are ready to begin cooking, gently heat 3 tbsp olive oil in a heavy-bottomed pot. Remove chicken portions, shallots or onions and mushrooms from the red-wine marinade (save this for later), place in the pot and cook until the meat is golden on both sides and the onions are translucent. Sprinkle flour over meat and stir until absorbed. Salt and pepper lightly. Add chicken stock and red-wine marinade; bring to a boil, then lower the heat and simmer, covered, for 40 minutes.

Meanwhile, heat 1 tablespoon olive oil in a skillet and cook the button mushrooms for 5-10 minutes until they have released some of their moisture. Add to the chicken and continue cooking until the chicken is tender, about 15 minutes.

Season to taste with salt and pepper, sprinkle with parsley, decorate with grapes and serve. Accompany with Bean mash (p. 188) or Pumpkin mash (p. 221) and a crisp green vegetable.

Chicken *gremolata*

This quick and easy recipe was inspired by *osso buco Milanese*, a delicious dish of veal shanks slowly braised in white wine. To me, the highlight of *osso buco* is the *gremolata*, a mixture of finely chopped parsley, lemon zest, anchovies and garlic that tastes profoundly of health, summer and the Mediterranean. I use chicken breasts when I'm in a hurry, but this works equally well with chicken thighs (which take longer to cook), with rabbit portions, turkey breast or tofu. Serves 4.

Warm the olive oil in a heavy-bottomed medium-sized pot. Dredge chicken lightly in the flour, shaking off any excess, and cook for 2-3 minutes on each side until golden; remove to a plate.

Pour stock and wine into the pot and scrape off any meat residues with a wooden spoon. Add chopped tomato, bay leaf and thyme and return chicken to the pot. Cook for 15 minutes, uncovered, to allow the sauce to thicken and the alcohol to evaporate. (If using thighs, cook for about 40 minutes, covered, at a gentle simmer.)

While the meat is cooking, prepare the *gremolata*: Finely chop parsley, garlic, anchovy and lemon zest with a *mezzaluna* herb chopper. Add to the sauce and cook for another minute or two until the anchovies have melted and the flavors have mingled thoroughly. Season with salt, pepper and perhaps a hint of honey to balance any excess acidity.

2 tbsp olive oil

1-1¼lb/500-600g skinless chicken breast

a little whole spelt/wheat flour for dusting

7fl oz/scant 1 cup/200ml chicken stock

3.5fl oz/scant ½ cup/100ml dry white wine

1 tomato, finely cubed

1 bay leaf

½ tsp thyme

acacia honey (optional)

salt & freshly ground black pepper

Gremolata

3 tbsp parsley, finely chopped

2 cloves garlic, finely chopped

1-2 canned anchovy fillets, rinsed and finely chopped

1 tbsp lemon zest (untreated)

Garlic, lemon and herb chicken kebabs

1.1lb/500g skinless chicken breast

2-3 cloves garlic, crushed

juice of ½ lemon

grated zest of ¼ lemon (untreated)

2-3 tbsp fresh and/or dried herbs (e.g. parsley, oregano, rosemary, sage)

1 tsp turmeric

3 tbsp olive oil

salt & freshly ground black pepper

1 red bell pepper, cut into 1-square-inch pieces

3.5oz/100g button mushrooms (halved if large)

4 lemon wedges as garnish

approx 10 metal, bamboo or wooden skewers

Here chicken breasts are infused with delightfully summery aromas of herbs, lemon, garlic and turmeric. It's fun to thread them on skewers, interspersed with peppers and mushrooms, and grilling them, but if you're pressed for time you can lightly sauté the marinated chicken pieces in olive oil (this yields child-friendly chicken "nuggets"). This works well with turkey or cubed tofu, too. Serves 4.

Cut the chicken breasts into bite-sized pieces and place in a bowl with a tight-fitting lid.

In a small blender, combine crushed garlic, lemon juice and zest, herbs, turmeric, olive oil and pepper. Blend into a smooth, creamy paste. Pour paste over chicken pieces and mix well so the meat is coated all over with the marinade. Do not add salt at this stage. Marinate for at least two hours in the refrigerator.

When you are ready to cook, preheat the grill to high setting. Thread meat, pepper pieces and mushrooms onto skewers and place on a wire grid placed in a grill pan to catch the juices. Slide skewers beneath grill and cook for about 10 minutes, turning frequently. The meat should be juicy but not pink at the center.

Lightly salt and serve with lemon wedges.

Chicken and apricot *tajine*

Named after the Moroccan clay dish in which these spicy stews were traditionally prepared, *tajines* are wonderfully versatile. Here I have replaced the more usual lamb with chicken, but this dish can also be made with rabbit or duck. You can either use dried fruit – apricots, prunes, figs, raisins or combinations of these – or fresh fruit, such as apples, pears or quinces, depending on the season. Serves 4.

Preheat oven to 350°F/180°C.

Warm 2 tablespoons olive oil in a large pot on medium heat and cook the chicken portions on both sides until golden; transfer to an ovenproof casserole dish.

In the remaining oil, cook the onions on medium heat until translucent (4-5 minutes). Add spices and cook for another minute, stirring so they don't burn. Add stock, stir and pour over the chicken pieces in the ovenproof dish, turning these over a few times so they are well coated. Cover with a lid and transfer to the oven.

After 40 minutes, remove lid and add apricots, submerging these in the cooking juices. Return to the oven for another 30 minutes, uncovered.

When the chicken pieces are cooked through, remove the dish from the oven and season with salt, pepper and lemon juice. Sprinkle with chopped walnuts and cilantro or parsley and serve. This is even better the next day when the flavors have had time to infuse.

3 tbsp olive oil

4 chicken thigh portions, or 1 small chicken cut into portions

2 onions, halved and sliced lengthwise

1 level tsp cinnamon

1 level tsp ground coriander

1 level tsp ground cumin

1 level tsp ground turmeric

1 level tsp ground cardamom

pinch of saffron strands or powder

5fl oz/⅔ cup/150ml chicken stock

3.5oz/100g apricots, pitted

squeeze of lemon juice

3 tbsp chopped walnuts

3 tbsp chopped cilantro or parsley

salt & freshly ground black pepper

Chicken *Marengo*

3 tbsp olive oil

1 small chicken cut into serving portions, or 4 chicken thigh portions

2 medium white onions, coarsely chopped

2 cloves garlic, finely chopped

pinch of mixed herbs (thyme, bay leaf, oregano)

1 tbsp whole wheat or spelt flour

3fl oz/⅓ cup/80ml white wine

3fl oz/⅓ cup/80ml chicken stock

15oz/400g tomatoes, fresh or from a jar

1.1lb/500g mushrooms

2 tbsp parsley, chopped

salt & freshly ground black pepper

Legend has it that French Emperor Napoleon Bonaparte first ate this dish after he defeated the Austrian army at Marengo, in the Piedmont region of Italy. He had not eaten before the battle and was ravenous. Alas, the foragers his cook sent out returned with meager findings: a scrawny chicken, four tomatoes, three eggs, a few crayfish, a little garlic and some olive oil. Napoleon's cook allegedly cut up the chicken with a saber and fried it in oil, crushed garlic and a little cognac filched from Napoleon's flask, together with the eggs and the crayfish. Over the years, the crayfish have been replaced with mushrooms and the eggs omitted altogether, leaving us with a succulent and simple chicken dish for all seasons and occasions. Serves 4.

In a heavy-bottomed pot, gently heat 2 tablespoons olive oil and cook the chicken pieces, turning them over occasionally until golden on all sides. Add onions, garlic and herbs. Cook another 3-4 minutes, stirring regularly. Sprinkle with flour and stir so the flour is well absorbed. Add wine, stock and tomatoes, cover and simmer on low heat for 40 minutes.

Meanwhile, cook mushrooms in 1 tablespoon olive oil on low heat for about 5 minutes. Add to the chicken and cook for another 10 minutes. Season with salt and pepper, sprinkle with parsley and serve.

Chicken couscous

This is a North African stew traditionally prepared with meat or fish and a variety of seasonal vegetables, legumes and warming spices. I've lightened it up a little by replacing the traditional mutton with chicken. Feel free to vary the vegetables to suit the seasons; green beans, cauliflower or zucchini work well too, for instance. Serve with quinoa couscous grain on p. 202. Serves 4.

In a heavy-bottomed pot, gently heat olive oil on medium heat and cook chicken pieces until golden on all sides. Remove and set aside.

Add onions to the pot and cook for another 3-4 minutes. Add spices and sauté with the onions, stirring, for another minute.

Pour in chicken stock and add garbanzos, carrots, turnips, fennel, celery and tomato paste. Return chicken portions, bring to the boil, cover and simmer on moderate heat. After 20 minutes, add squash and cabbage and cook, uncovered, another 10 minutes or until chicken is done. Remove chicken skin and discard; return chicken portions to stew.

Season with salt, pepper and lemon juice and sprinkle withchopped cilantro or parsley. I have kept this stew intentionally mild, but if you want it to taste more authentic, serve it with *harissa*, a spicy North African paste made of chili peppers, garlic and spices.

Ras el hanout *is a Moroccan spice mix that usually includes nutmeg, ginger, pepper, aniseed, cumin, cardamom, chillies, turmeric, cloves, cinnamon, paprika, cayenne and allspice. To make your own, use* ½ *tsp turmeric,* ½ *tsp coriander,* ¼ *tsp ground ginger,* ¼ *tsp cinnamon,* ¼ *tsp cumin and* ¼ *tsp paprika powder to replace two teaspoons* ras el hanout.

---

2 tbsp olive oil

1-1½kg chicken, cut into portions

2 onions, chopped

2 tsp ras el hanout (see below)

2 tsp cinnamon

2 pints/1l chicken stock

15oz/400g cooked garbanzos

4 carrots, chopped into thirds

2-3 turnips, coarsely cubed

1 bulb fennel, sliced

2 ribs celery, cubed

2 tbsp tomato paste

15oz/400g Hokkaido squash or sweet potato chopped into ½-inch cubes

9oz/250 g kale, Savoy cabbage or broccoli, coarsely chopped

squeeze of lemon juice

salt and pepper to taste

2 tbsp chopped cilantro or parsley

Rabbit in mustard sauce

1 tbsp olive oil

1 rabbit (about 2.5-3lb/1.2 kg), cut into portions

2 large onions, quartered and thinly sliced

½ tsp thyme

7fl oz/1 scant cup/200ml dry white wine

1 heaped tbsp coarse mustard

1 heaped tbsp smooth (e.g. Dijon) mustard

3.5fl oz/scant ½ cup/100ml Cashew cream (see p. 231)

squeeze of lemon juice

salt & freshly ground black pepper

1 tbsp chopped parsley

This classic French country recipe suits all seasons and is very easy to prepare. Slowly braising the rabbit in the oven on a bed of onions keeps the meat moist and succulent (being very lean, rabbit meat dries out easily when grilled or baked on its own). If you don't like the idea of eating rabbit, you can substitute it with chicken. Serves 4.

Preheat oven to 350°F/180°C.

In a large ovenproof pot on medium heat, gently cook rabbit portions in olive oil until golden on both sides. Remove to a plate and cook onions and thyme in the remaining olive oil until soft, stirring regularly.

Add white wine and mustards and mix with the onions until evenly distributed. Return rabbit portions to the pot, coating it on all sides with the onion-mustard mixture. Bring back to a gentle simmer, cover tightly and place in the preheated oven. Bake for 1 hour.

When ready, remove from oven and gently stir Cashew cream into the onion-mustard paste. Season to taste with salt, pepper and lemon juice and sprinkle with freshly chopped parsley. Serve with a green vegetable (e.g. spinach, Swiss chard, asparagus, green beans) and Bean mash (p. 188) or Pumpkin mash (p. 221).

Italian rabbit stew

In this versatile recipe, feel free to vary the vegetables according to the season. If you don't like rabbit or have trouble obtaining it, it can easily be replaced with chicken portions. Serves 4.

Combine the first nine ingredients in a large container with a tight-fitting lid. Add the rabbit portions and mix thoroughly to ensure they're well-coated. Marinate overnight in the refrigerator. (If you don't have time for this, start from scratch on the day you're eating this; it'll still be very tasty.)

When you're ready to cook, preheat oven to 350°F/180°C.

In a large pot, warm the olive oil and gently cook the rabbit portions until golden on all sides. Now pour over the marinade (wine, onions, garlic, carrots, celery, capers and herbs), add mushrooms and slowly bring to a boil.

Cover with a tight-fitting lid and place in the oven to stew for ½ hour. Add tomatoes and cook another ½ hour. Remove from oven, season to taste with salt and pepper, freshly grated lemon zest and lemon juice. (*Gremolata* works well too.)

Serve with Bean mash (p. 188), Garlicky spinach (p. 220) or any other seasonal vegetable.

1 onion, finely sliced

4 spring onions, left whole

2 ribs celery, coarsely chopped

2 carrots, coarsely chopped

3-4 cloves garlic, thinly sliced

1 tsp capers, rinsed of their brine

½ tsp each of thyme, rosemary and oregano

2 bay leaves

7fl oz/scant 1 cup/200ml white wine

1 rabbit (about 2.5-3lb/1.2 kg), cut into portions

3 tbsp olive oil

3.5oz/100g chestnut or porcini mushrooms or 1oz/25g dried, rehydrated mushrooms

3 tomatoes, coarsely chopped

zest and juice of ½ lemon

salt & freshly ground black pepper

Beans and legumes

Throughout the Mediterranean region, beans and legumes have been a dietary staple for thousands of years, essential for supplementing protein whenever meat or fish were scarce. Legumes also provide a broad range of minerals and vitamins, antioxidant plant nutrients and phytoestrogens.

Most beans are available in jars, pre-cooked and ready to use. However, conserved beans can't quite match the flavor or texture of beans cooked from scratch, so you may want to soak and cook them yourself when you can find a little extra time. In the recipes that follow I simply refer to "cooked" legumes; it's up to you to decide whether to buy them in jars or to soak and cook them yourself – both are fine.

When soaking and cooking legumes from scratch, begin by picking through them and removing any stones, broken beans or other debris. Transfer to a large bowl, cover with drinking-quality water and remove "floaters."

I recommend 12 hours' soaking time; this is best done overnight. Soaking and cooking roughly doubles the weight of dried legumes; thus 3.5 ounces/100 grams dry beans yields about 7 ounces/200 grams rehydrated beans.

When you are ready to cook the soaked beans, tip them into a strainer and rinse thoroughly. Transfer them to a large, heavy-bottomed pot, cover with cold water and bring to the boil. Then turn down the heat and let the beans simmer gently until soft. Skim off any foam that rises to the surface. Add seasonings such as or onions, garlic, bay leaf and thyme. Savory also goes very well with legumes and makes them easier to digest.

About halfway through the cooking time, when the beans have begun to soften, you can add salt and any acidic ingredients like tomatoes. Cooking times depend on the freshness of the beans (the older the beans, the longer they take to soften), but start checking after about 45 minutes.

I often soak and cook more beans than I need for a specific recipe and freeze the rest in sealable bags. That way, I always have ready-to-use legumes to hand that can be rapidly defrosted.

Warm Puy lentil, carrot & hazelnut salad

This lukewarm salad can be enjoyed throughout the year, especially in late winter when local salad greens and vegetables become rather uninspiring. Feel free to add other herbs such as chives or basil, maybe a pinch of lemon zest, different nuts (walnuts and walnut oil perhaps), crumbled cheese (e.g. feta) and even cubes of a tart apple (e.g. Granny Smith). Serves 4.

Preheat oven to 350°F/180°C.

Tip soaked lentils into a pot, cover with plenty of water and bring to the boil. Once boiling, reduce heat, cover and simmer until the lentils are soft but *al dente*, about 15 minutes.

Meanwhile, scatter hazelnuts on a baking tray, slide into the oven and toast for 10 minutes. Remove and cool. Once cooled, tip onto a clean tea towel, fold towel over and rub nuts together to remove as much as possible of their skins. Chop coarsely.

Next, mix vinegar, oils and garlic in a wide serving bowl. Add onion and carrot to the dressing. Once the lentils are cooked, strain them into a sieve and tip into salad bowl.

Quickly mix everything together and allow vegetables to warm through. Taste again for seasoning – you may need to add extra vinegar and salt. Scatter with chopped parsley and nuts.

Variation

This tastes delicious with fresh goats' cheese or feta cheese crumbled over it.

9 oz/1¼ cup/250g dry French green lentils, soaked for at least 8 hours

2oz/50g whole hazelnuts

3 tbsp balsamic vinegar

3 tbsp olive oil (or a mix of olive and hazelnut oil)

1 large or 2 small cloves garlic, crushed

½ red onion, finely chopped

3 carrots, peeled and grated

3 tbsp flat-leaf parsley, coarsely chopped

salt & freshly ground black pepper

Bean mash

2fl oz/¼ cup/60ml olive oil

3 sprigs fresh rosemary (or 2 tsp dried rosemary)

6 cloves garlic, finely sliced

5-6 chopped sage leaves

1.3lb/2⅔ cups/600g cooked navy beans

2fl oz/¼ cup/60ml water or vegetable stock

zest of ½ lemon (untreated)

squeeze of lemon juice

salt & freshly ground black pepper

If you love mashed potatoes but worry about their glycemic impact, help is at hand with this delicious dish. Beans offer the same starchy texture as floury potatoes but they're a vastly superior source of protein, fiber and low-glycemic carbohydrates. Being bland tasting, they are an excellent vehicle for the heady aromas of rosemary, sage, garlic, lemon and olive oil. Serves 4 as a side dish.

In a heavy-bottomed pot, gently warm three quarters of the olive oil with 2 rosemary sprigs (or 2 teaspoons dry rosemary) on medium heat. When it sizzles, remove pan from heat and infuse rosemary for 10 minutes.

Remove rosemary (if using dry rosemary, remove as much as you can with a small strainer or spoon) and add garlic to the oil, return to low heat and cook gently for 30-40 seconds. Add sage leaves, beans and water or stock and stir. Cook for 10 minutes on low heat and remove.

With a potato masher or an electric hand-held blender, roughly mash the beans in the pot until you obtain a thick paste. If it's too thick, add hot water a tablespoon at a time until you achieve the desired consistency.

Grate lemon zest into the puree, season to taste with salt, pepper and lemon juice. Just before serving, drizzle remaining olive oil on top and stir lightly. Decorate with a fresh sprig of rosemary and serve immediately.

Variations
- Combine the beans with chopped or pureed roasted red bell peppers for added flavor and color.
- ½ tsp turmeric adds a golden glow.
- If you prefer the texture of whole beans, skip the mashing stage.

Lentil moussaka

This dish is inspired by the famous Greek *Moussaka me melitzanes*, but the name is where the similarity ends. First, I have replaced fatty lamb with nutty French green lentils. Secondly, I do not sauté the eggplant slices in oil, but brush them lightly with olive oil and grill them, thus using much less fat and lightening up the dish. Serves 4-6.

Warm 2 tablespoons of the oil in a large pot on medium heat and gently cook onions and garlic until translucent (about 4-5 minutes). Add herbs and cinnamon, tomatoes, mushrooms and red wine and cook uncovered for 20 minutes until reduced by about one third; puree with a hand-held blender. Add cooked lentils to the tomato sauce and cook for another 15 minutes. Remove from heat.

While the lentil sauce is cooking, lightly brush both sides of the eggplant slices with olive oil and place on a baking tray covered with baking parchment. Set grill on medium heat and grill eggplant slices on both sides until golden. Set aside.

For the *béchamel* topping, put cold milk, 3 tablespoons olive oil, flour, turmeric and nutmeg in a pot and whisk until combined. Set over medium heat and stir. After 2-3 minutes the mixture will start thickening; keep stirring until it bubbles gently. Cook another 1-2 minutes, stirring all the while. Remove from heat.

Lightly oil an ovenproof dish and get ready to layer. Start with a thin layer of lentil-tomato sauce followed by a layer of eggplant and continue in this way until you end with lentils on top.

Finish by pouring the *béchamel* over the pie and smoothing it out evenly with a spatula. Place in a preheated oven and cook for 15 minutes; sprinkle with crumbled feta cheese and cook another 10 minutes until the cheese is golden. Serve.

2fl oz/¼ cup/60ml olive oil plus 3 tbsp

2 onions, sliced

2 cloves garlic, chopped

2 bay leaves

½ tsp thyme

1 tsp each of oregano and mint

1 tsp cinnamon

1¾ lb/800g tomatoes, cubed

1oz/25g dried porcini or shiitake mushrooms, rehydrated, drained and finely chopped

3.5fl oz/½ cup/120ml red wine

1.3lb/2⅔ cups/600 g cooked French green lentils

3 large eggplants cut into 6-7 mm slices

13.5fl oz/1⅔ cups/400ml unsweetened soy or almond milk

3 tbsp whole wheat or spelt flour

1 tsp turmeric

pinch of grated nutmeg

salt & pepper

3.5 oz/100 g feta cheese

Falafel with sesame dip

1 medium onion

3 tbsp parsley leaves

3 tbsp cilantro leaves

3-4 cloves garlic, crushed

1 tsp ground coriander

1 tsp ground cumin

1 tsp turmeric

pinch of lemon zest (untreated)

15oz/400g cooked garbanzos

2 tbsp whole wheat or spelt flour

2 tbsp ground flax seeds

1 tsp baking powder

1 egg

salt & black pepper

4-5 tbsp olive oil

Sesame dip

1 clove garlic, crushed

3 tbsp tahini (sesame paste)

juice of ½ lemon

pinch of lemon zest

5-6 tbsp water

salt & black pepper

These nutty garbanzo balls from the Eastern Mediterranean delight vegetarians and meat-eaters alike. Serve them Mid-East-style in warmed wholegrain pita pockets with shredded salad, onions, tomatoes, cabbage and sesame dip (below), enjoy them on a plate accompanied by mixed salad and/or a cooked vegetable, or serve as finger-food at aperitif time. Serves 4.

Coarsely chop onion and herbs, place in a food processor with crushed garlic, spices and lemon zest and whizz until the herbs and onions are finely chopped. Add garbanzos, flour, baking powder, ground flax seed and egg and pulse briefly until you get a ball of sticky dough. Season to taste with salt and pepper, and leave to rest for 30 minutes.

Heat olive oil in a large skillet. Using a teaspoon, form walnut-sized balls of dough that you place carefully in the hot pan, slightly flattening them with a spatula. Cook until golden on one side (2-3 minutes) and turn over, cooking until golden. Lift falafels out of the pan and drain excess fat on a paper towel. Serve immediately with sesame dip.

For the sesame dip, place all the ingredients (except water) in a small blender and whizz until you obtain a smooth, creamy emulsion. Add water to achieve the desired texture. Season to taste with salt and pepper and serve alongside falafels. This sauce also tastes great drizzled over crisp green vegetables such as broccoli or green beans.

Greek bean stew

This hearty stew is inspired by Greece's *fassolatha*, a bean-and-vegetable dish that was traditionally eaten during Lent when meat was forbidden for religious reasons. A rich blend of creamy beans, chunky vegetables, sweet tomato and velvety olive oil makes this a comforting and nourishing dish. In Greece, *fassolatha* is eaten warm or at room temperature and is traditionally served with feta cheese (Marinated feta cheese, p. 121), crusty bread and black olives. Serves 4.

In a large, heavy-bottomed pot, warm the olive oil and cook chopped onion and garlic until translucent (4-5 minutes). Add carrots, celery and sweet potato cubes and continue cooking, stirring well, for 5 minutes.

Add beans, dry herbs and stock, bring to the boil, reduce heat and cover. Cook until all vegetables are soft (15-20 minutes). Add tomato paste and cook for another 5 minutes.

With a hand-held blender, briefly whizz the stew three to four times to create a thicker texture, but not to the point of obtaining a puree (unless that's what you want).

Remove from heat and add grated lemon zest. Season to taste with salt, pepper and lemon juice and sprinkle with chopped fresh herbs. Serve warm, handing around marinated feta cheese and olives for everyone to serve themselves.

2 tbsp olive oil

1 large onion, chopped

3 cloves garlic, finely chopped

4 carrots, peeled and thinly sliced

2 ribs celery, cubed

1 medium sweet potato, peeled and finely cubed

1.1lb/500g cooked navy beans

generous pinch each of dried savory or thyme and oregano

2 pints/1l vegetable stock

3 tbsp tomato paste

pinch of lemon zest

squeeze of lemon juice

2 tbsp chopped fresh herbs (e.g. parsley, oregano or mint)

salt & freshly ground black pepper

a portion Marinated feta cheese (p. 121)

Hummus

15oz/400g cooked garbanzos, drained

2 tbsp olive oil

juice of 1 lemon

pinch of lemon zest (untreated)

1 clove garlic, crushed

5 fl oz/⅔ cup/150 ml water or garbanzo cooking liquid

3oz/⅓ cup/80g tahini (sesame paste)

olive oil and red pepper flakes or paprika powder as garnish

salt & freshly ground black pepper

This tasty Eastern Mediterranean garbanzo and sesame puree is a powerhouse of nutrition, supplying protein, fiber, phytoestrogens, garlic and healthy fats. It makes a delicious dip for raw vegetables, a succulent sandwich filling (topped, for example, with broccoli sprouts or grilled bell peppers) or a speedy *hors d'oeuvre* served in an avocado half. This is a basic hummus recipe; you can add chopped, grilled red bell peppers or beet cubes for an orange or pink hue and/or sprinkle with chopped olives or toasted pine nuts for garnish. Makes about 1.1lb/500g.

Drain the softened garbanzos but reserve cooking liquid. Place garbanzos in a food processor with olive oil, lemon juice and zest, garlic and water (if you've soaked and cooked the garbanzos from scratch, use the cooking liquid). Start blending and gradually add tahini. The consistency should be like thick cream; if it seems too dry, add more cooking liquid or water.

Season to taste with salt and pepper. Transfer to a serving bowl, drizzle with olive oil and sprinkle with red pepper flakes or paprika powder.

Tofu

Tofu is a protein-rich, cream-colored food that is produced by coagulating soy milk (made from soy beans) and then pressing the resulting curds into blocks. It is used in many Asian cuisines and is popular among vegetarians and vegans in the west.

As discussed earlier, it is not clear to what extent soy foods are cancer-protective; while some research indicates that the phytoestrogens in soy may decrease certain risks, other studies don't bear this out. The answer is likely complex and may depend on a person's age, health status, the age at which they began eating soy foods, and even the presence or absence of specific bacteria in their digestive tract.

However, eaten in moderation and in the form of traditional soy-based foods such as tofu, rather than as highly processed meat imitations or convenience-food additives, soy deserves a place in a varied healthy diet and can be a useful alternative protein source to meat and fish. Fermented soy foods, such as tempeh, natto and miso, are thought to be particularly beneficial as they are easier to assimilate and provide a useful source of healthy bacteria. Moreover, fermentation is thought to make soy isoflavones more biovailable to humans.

Tofu has a bland, almost chalky flavor, which on its own isn't terribly enticing. However, it gratefully absorbs the rich aromas of many Mediterranean preparations, especially those involving tomatoes, garlic, onions, mustard or lemon.

Soy bean curd comes in a range of textures, ranging from firm square or rectangular blocks to smooth "silken" tofu whose texture resembles that of a light egg custard. It is sold refrigerated or non-refrigerated in sealed packs. Once the packages are opened, all types of tofu should be rinsed, kept in a container covered with water, chilled and used within a few days.

Avocado, tomato and tofu *tricolora*

3.5oz/100g firm tofu, sliced and marinated overnight in 2 tbsp basil pesto (p. 229)

2oz/50 g pine nuts

3-4 firm tomatoes

1 ripe but firm avocado

olive oil

1 tbsp balsamic vinegar

15 basil leaves, roughly torn or shredded

salt & freshly ground black pepper

Inspired by Italy's *insalata tricolora* (tomatoes, mozzarella and basil), this light *hors d'oeuvre* brims with summer aromas: spicy tomatoes, sweet basil, fruity olive oil, fragrant balsamic vinegar and nutty pine nuts. The innovation is tofu instead of mozzarella. Serves 4.

Slice tofu into ¼-inch/5mm slices and place in a container with a lid. Add pesto (perhaps diluted with a little water to make it runnier) and combine, ensuring that the tofu is well coated with the pesto. Seal and refrigerate for several hours, ideally overnight.

When you are ready to prepare the salad, toast pine nuts in a dry pan on low heat until golden and fragrant (2-3 minutes). Transfer to a bowl to cool.

Slice the tomatoes with a sharp knife, taking care to remove the fibrous core. Halve the avocado, remove the stone, halve again, peel quarters carefully and slice.

Arrange tomatoes, avocado and marinated tofu on a large serving plate. Drizzle with olive oil and balsamic vinegar, scatter with pine nuts and basil leaves and season lightly with salt and freshly ground black pepper. Serve immediately.

Tofu in red wine sauce

Inspired by the classic French beef stew, *boeuf bourguignon*, this is a tasty way of eating tofu. Serves 4 .

To make the marinade, combine red wine, garlic, tamari, thyme leaves and chopped onion in a container with a tight-fitting lid. Add tofu cubes, coat with the marinade, close lid and chill for at least one hour, or preferably overnight.

When ready to cook, warm 2 tablespoons oil in a heavy-bottomed pot. Strain off the marinade (reserve this) and cook tofu, onions and garlic in the pot. Stir occasionally so that the tofu browns on all sides (about 10 minutes). Sprinkle with flour and stir well until it is completely absorbed.

Add marinade and stock and stir well. Add carrots, bring to boil and then lower heat and cook, uncovered, for 20 minutes, or until soft.

Meanwhile in a skillet, warm remaining 2 tablespoons olive oil and sauté mushrooms. Cook on medium heat until all excess moisture has evaporated and the mushrooms have reduced in size. Add to pot along with tomato paste and simmer for another 5 minutes. Remove from heat, season with salt and pepper and garnish with chopped parsley.

10fl oz/1 ¼ cups/300ml red wine

2 cloves garlic, chopped

2 tbsp tamari (wheat-free soy sauce)

½ tsp thyme

1 large onion, finely chopped

1.1lb/500g plain, firm tofu, cut into 1 cm cubes

4 tbsp olive oil

2 tbsp whole wheat, spelt or corn flour

7fl oz/scant 1 cup/200ml vegetable stock

3-4 carrots, peeled and sliced

15oz/400g button mushrooms, quartered

1 tbsp tomato paste

salt & freshly ground black pepper

2 tbsp chopped parsley

Tofu *Dijonnaise*

3 tbsp olive oil

2 tbsp lemon juice

finely grated zest of ½ untreated lemon

2oz/50g mustard (half whole-grain, half Dijon-style)

3 cloves garlic, crushed

1 tbsp fresh rosemary, coarsely chopped

15oz/400g firm, plain tofu, cut into ½-inch/1cm cubes

3.5fl oz/scant ½ cup/100ml dry white wine

3.5fl oz/scant ½ cup/100ml Cashew cream (p. 231)

1 tbsp parsley, chopped

salt & freshly ground black pepper

Mustard, a member of the Brassica family, is a great way of infusing tofu with taste, assisted here by lemon juice and zest, garlic and rosemary – a classic Mediterranean blend of flavors. For best results, marinate tofu overnight. Serves 4.

In a sealable container, combine olive oil, lemon juice and zest, mustard, garlic, rosemary, salt and pepper and stir well to mix. Add cubed tofu, close lid and refrigerate for at least 3 hours, ideally overnight.

When you are ready to cook, warm a large skillet and tip in the marinated tofu. Cook for 10-12 minutes, stirring every 3-4 minutes until cubes are browned on all sides.

Add white wine and marinade and bring to the boil. Now add Cashew cream and stir until the sauce thickens. Remove from heat, season with salt, pepper and lemon juice, sprinkle with parsley and serve immediately.

Variation
This recipe is also delicious with chicken breasts, cut into large chunks, marinated and cooked the same way.

Moroccan tofu

This recipe's complex blend of spices, herbs and nuts, yielding an amazingly sweet-yet-spicy flavor, belies the utter simplicity of its preparation. (This recipe also works well using cubed chicken breast instead of tofu.) Serve with Saffron quinoa (p. 202) and crisp, green vegetables. Serves 4.

Begin by marinating the tofu: in a container with a tight-fitting lid, mix 1 tablespoon olive oil, turmeric, *ras el hanout*, lemon juice, ground black pepper and 1 clove crushed garlic into a paste. Cube tofu, add to spice paste and stir until coated. Cover and chill, ideally overnight.

Begin preparing the dish by gently toasting the chopped almonds in a dry skillet. Cook for 2-3 minutes, stirring, until golden and fragrant. Remove to a plate and set aside to cool.

Next, heat 1 tablespoon olive oil in the skillet on medium heat and add tofu. Cook gently and turn cubes with a spatula every 4-5 minutes until golden on all sides; this should take about 10-15 minutes.

While the tofu is cooking, warm the remaining olive oil in a pot and cook chopped garlic, ginger and chili or paprika. Add tomatoes, saffron and cinnamon and continue cooking for 10 minutes, stirring regularly. Season with salt, pepper and honey.

Stir golden tofu cubes into the tomato sauce, sprinkle with crunchy almonds and chopped parsley or cilantro and serve immediately.

---

3 tbsp olive oil

½ tsp turmeric

½ tsp ras el hanout *(see p. 183)*

juice of ½ lemon

7 cloves garlic, 1 crushed and 6 chopped

15 oz/400g plain, firm tofu

2 tbsp almonds, chopped

1 inch/2cm fresh ginger, peeled and finely chopped

pinch of chili flakes or paprika powder

1¾ lb/800g tomatoes, roughly cubed

1 generous pinch saffron

½ tsp cinnamon

1-2 tbsp honey (to taste)

salt & freshly ground black pepper

2-3 tbsp parsley or cilantro, chopped

1 tbsp olive oil

Tofu and vegetable cabbage parcels

1 Savoy cabbage, dark outer leaves removed

1 onion

2 carrots

2 cloves garlic, crushed

1 rib celery

3.5oz/100g button mushrooms

10oz/300g firm tofu

1 tbsp olive oil

¼ tsp thyme

1 tbsp chopped chives

1 tbsp chopped parsley

1 large egg, lightly beaten

salt and pepper

9fl oz/1 cup/250ml Basic tomato sauce (p. 226)

Cabbage leaves are often stuffed with a ground meat, which we replace here with tofu and finely chopped vegetables. This dish is especially tasty when the cabbage rolls are baked in tomato sauce but if you're pressed for time, just chop a few fresh tomatoes into the dish, lightly salt and pepper these and place cabbage parcels on top. Serves 4.

Preheat oven to 350°F/180°C.

Bring a large pot of water to the boil and salt. With a sharp knife, cut 12-14 large leaves off the cabbage, place these in the boiling water and blanch for 3 minutes until soft but not wilted. Drain and rinse with cold running water. Set aside.

Finely chop vegetables (onion, carrots, garlic, celery, mushrooms and remaining cabbage) and tofu. Heat olive oil in a large skillet and cook vegetables and tofu for 5 minutes, stirring gently from time to time. Add herbs and stir. Remove from heat and cool for 5 minutes before adding beaten egg. Season with salt and pepper.

Place cooled cabbage leaves flat on a work surface and fill them with the tofu-and-vegetable stuffing. Roll up, first the sides, then lengthways, and secure with a wooden cocktail stick or tie with kitchen string.

Pour tomato sauce in an ovenproof gratin dish, place the cabbage parcels on top, cover with foil and cook in a medium oven for 40 minutes until the cabbage is soft.

Whole grains, pizza, pasta

Grain-based dishes have traditionally been a popular source of energy and nutrition around the Mediterranean. Not only wheat but also buckwheat (which, despite its name, is not a member of the wheat family and does not contain gluten), rye and spelt – sometimes enriched with added sesame or flax seeds – were widely consumed.

Before the Mediterranean region became industrialized and most people led physically tiring lives as peasants or artisans, a high intake of carbohydrates from grains may have been useful. However, people with largely sedentary western lifestyles need to be careful not to eat too many grain-based meals, especially when the grains are refined.

Not only are these less nutrient-rich than other plant foods such as vegetables, fruits or nuts, they can also have adverse effects on our blood-sugar balance and our waistline. Moreover, allergies or intolerances to gluten-containing grains are common, another reason to limit their consumption.

This is not to say that we should never eat cereal grains; however, when we do, we should be very choosy about the types of grain products we eat, favoring whole, unprocessed, organically grown grains and varying these as much as possible. Moreover, in many cases, soaking, sprouting and fermentation – for example, through the use of sourdough – makes grains more nutritious and easier to digest.

In many of the recipes that follow, I have reproduced classic Mediterranean grain dishes but have exchanged many traditional cereal and flour products with gluten-free alternatives. Thus, couscous semolina is substituted with quinoa, a gluten-free, protein-rich South American grain; pizza dough is made with almonds and flax seeds instead of flour; and spaghetti is replaced – when in season – with spaghetti squash.

Meanwhile, in the more traditional pasta dishes that follow, I recommend using wholegrain pasta, which may include spelt or kamut as a change from wheat.

"Pizza"

For the pizza base

3.5oz/100g golden flax seeds, finely ground in a coffee grinder

3.5oz/100g finely ground almonds

pinch of herbes de Provence

1 tsp baking powder

½ tsp salt

4 eggs

1 clove garlic, crushed

4 tbsp olive oil

5fl oz/ ⅔ cup/150ml water

No Mediterranean cookbook would be complete without a pizza recipe. Here I propose a dish that looks like pizza, smells like pizza and tastes (almost) like pizza – but that contains neither wheat nor yeast and is a tasty way of integrating lignin-rich flax seeds into your diet. This light and airy base will accommodate any toppings you would find on conventional pizza; my favorites are a layer of Basic tomato sauce (p. 226) covered with thinly sliced zucchini, sliced mushrooms, chopped artichoke hearts, thinly sliced onions, drained sardines, anchovies or tuna, olives, capers or thinly sliced bell peppers. Serves 4.

Preheat the oven to 350°F/180°C. Cover a baking tray (about 12 by 16 inches/30 by 40 cm) with a sheet of baking parchment.

In a mixing bowl, combine ground flax seeds, ground almonds, herbs, baking powder and salt. In another mixing bowl, beat eggs, crushed garlic, olive oil and water together. Pour the liquid mixture over the dry ingredients and whisk to obtain a smooth paste. Spread this onto the baking tray and slide into the oven. Bake for about 20-25 minutes, until golden on top.

Remove from the oven, cool for 5 minutes, then tip upside down onto a second baking tray (or onto a chopping board and slide, upside down, back onto the tray you were using before). The base is now ready to be garnished.

Increase oven temperature to 400°F/200°C. Once you have garnished the base with toppings of your choice, return to the oven for 10 minutes until toppings are cooked. Serve immediately.

Pissaladière

For this healthy take on *pissaladière*, the famous onion pizza from the French Mediterranean town of Nice, sweet caramelized onions with a hint of capery sharpness are slathered onto the flax-and-almond pizza base on the opposite page and topped with anchovies and black olives. Serves 4.

Preheat the oven to 350°F/180°C.

In a large, heavy-bottomed skillet on medium heat, warm olive oil and cook onions, garlic, thyme and bay leaf with a light sprinkling of salt and pepper. Cover and stir frequently to prevent sticking.

Cook until softened – about ½ hour. If there is too much moisture, remove lid and let juices evaporate for 5-10 minutes; the onion mixture should be creamy but not wet. Drain capers, chop finely and stir into softened onions.

While the onions are cooking, prepare pizza base as described in the "Pizza" recipe on the previous page. Bake until golden. Remove pastry base from the oven and evenly spread softened onions over it. Now lay the anchovy fillets on top in a crisscross grid-pattern, placing a black olive at every intersection of anchovy fillets.

Return *pissaladière* to the oven and bake for 10 minutes until the onions are golden. Serve hot, with an accompaniment of lightly dressed mixed salad leaves or a crunchy green vegetable such as broccoli or green beans.

1 almond-flax pizza base (see previous page)

Topping

4 tbsp olive oil

2lb/1kg onions, peeled, halved and finely sliced

3 cloves garlic, finely chopped

½ tsp thyme

1 bay leaf

1 tbsp capers, rinsed in water

12 anchovy fillets packed in olive oil in a jar

10-15 black olives

salt & freshly ground black pepper

Quinoa couscous

2 tbsp olive oil

1 small onion, finely chopped

7oz/1 cup/200g dry quinoa, thoroughly rinsed

13½ fl oz/1⅔ cups/400ml vegetable or chicken stock

1 stick cinnamon

1 tbsp unsalted butter

2 tbsp sultanas

2 tbsp almond slivers

salt to taste

To accompany chicken couscous or similar north African stews, I suggest you commit the heresy of replacing the traditional wheat semolina (delicious, but with a fairly high GI rating) with protein-rich, nutty quinoa, prepared here just like traditional couscous with raisins, almonds and a little melted butter. Serves 4 as a side dish.

In a heavy-bottomed pot on medium heat, warm olive oil and cook onion until translucent (4-5 minutes). Add quinoa and stir until well coated with oil. Add stock and cinnamon stick. Bring to the boil, cover and simmer on lowest possible setting for 20 minutes or until grains have absorbed all the stock and are easily fluffed up with a fork.

Once cooked, remove from heat and add butter, sultanas and almond slivers. Stir lightly with a fork to combine butter and grains without creating lumps. Season with salt and serve. Leftovers are delicious for breakfast drizzled with warm almond milk and a little honey.

Saffron quinoa

2 tbsp olive oil

1 onion, chopped

2 cloves garlic, chopped

7oz/1 cup/200g dry quinoa, thoroughly rinsed

13½ fl oz/1⅔ cups/400ml chicken or vegetable stock

pinch of saffron

salt & freshly ground black pepper

Here, garlic, onions and saffron soften quinoa's slightly chalky taste by adding a touch of sweetness and a beautiful golden glow.

In a heavy-bottomed pot on medium heat, warm olive oil and gently cook onion and garlic, stirring regularly, for 4-5 minutes or until translucent. Add quinoa and stir thoroughly to coat the grains with the oil.

Add stock and saffron and bring to the boil. Cover, reduce heat and cook on lowest setting for 20 minutes or until grains have absorbed all the stock and are easily fluffed up with a fork. Once the quinoa is cooked, remove from heat and serve. Can be garnished with crunchy almonds and chopped parsley for added texture and visual appeal.

Pasta in a garlicky olive-oil dressing

Spaghetti aglio e olio has got to be one of the simplest, speediest and tastiest pasta dishes of all time. Garlic, pepper flakes, olive oil, anchovies and pine nuts provide delicious cancer-protective nutrients while a dusting of Parmesan lifts protein content and flavor. Serves 4.

Toast pine nuts in a small, dry skillet on medium heat for 2-3 minutes until they start to turn a light golden color and give off a nutty, baked fragrance. Transfer to a plate and reserve.

In a large pot, boil salted water and cook spaghetti according to the instructions on the package.

While the pasta is cooking, finely chop garlic. In a deep, heavy-bottomed skillet, heat 2 tablespoons olive oil and cook anchovies for 2 minutes until they turn soft and start to come apart. Add garlic and pepper flakes and cook for another 30 seconds. Remove from heat and set aside until the pasta is *al dente*.

Drain pasta and tip into the pan containing the garlicky oil; drizzle with remaining oil, toss carefully, season with salt and pepper, sprinkle with pine nuts, dust with grated cheese and serve.

Variations
- To boost protein content, add cooked meat or fish leftovers.
- Add chopped olives or sun-dried tomatoes with the garlic.
- In summer, fresh chopped tomatoes stirred into the hot pasta just before serving are delicious.
- Add fresh herbs such as basil and oregano leaves.
- For a quick and tasty vegetable side-dish, replace pasta with crisply steamed green beans.

---

2 tbsp pine nuts

15oz/400g whole grain spaghetti

5 cloves garlic

5-6 tbsp olive oil

4 anchovy fillets in olive oil, rinsed

1 tsp dried red pepper flakes or finely chopped fresh chili

2 tbsp finely grated Parmesan or pecorino cheese

salt & freshly ground black pepper

Spaghetti *puttanesca*

4 tbsp olive oil

pinch of red pepper flakes

2 cloves garlic, chopped

2oz/50g anchovies in olive oil, rinsed

15oz/400g tomatoes, chopped

1-2 tbsp capers, rinsed

3.5oz/100g black olives

2 tbsp tomato paste

15oz/400g whole grain spaghetti or other pasta shapes

2 tbsp chopped parsley

salt & freshly ground black pepper

This famous Italian store-cupboard classic featuring tomatoes, olive and capers is super quick, super nourishing and delicious! Serves 4.

In a large pot, boil water for the pasta.

Pour olive oil into a skillet, add red pepper flakes and garlic and cook for 1 minute, stirring constantly. Add anchovies and keep stirring. Add tomatoes, capers, olives and tomato paste and cook for 15 minutes on medium heat. Season sparingly with salt (the olives, capers and anchovies are salty already) and pepper.

Once the water is boiling, add salt and pasta and cook *al dente*. When they are ready, drain the spaghetti in a strainer and tip into the tomato sauce, tossing well to coat the pasta with the sauce.

Sprinkle with chopped parsley and serve.

Lentil Bolognese with spaghetti squash

This is an unusual vegetarian take on Italy's most famous meaty pasta sauce. Spaghetti squash makes a tasty alternative to pasta, but when this is not in season, you can serve this sauce atop pasta or use as a filling for lasagna. Serves 4.

Cut the raw squash in two halves, scrape out seeds and steam in a large pot, flesh facing upward. Test for doneness after 30 minutes: the squash is ready when the flesh can be pulled out with a fork in spaghetti-like threads cooked *al dente*. Scrape flesh carefully into a warmed serving bowl, season with salt and pepper, drizzle with 2 tablespoons olive oil, toss gently, cover and keep warm.

While the squash is being steamed, heat olive oil in a pot and cook onion and garlic until translucent. Add carrot, leek, celery and mushrooms and cook, stirring, for 10 minutes. Add lentils, herbs, red wine and milk and reduce by half.

Add tomatoes and tomato paste, cover and cook for another 10 minutes. Season with salt and pepper; if the tomatoes are sour, add a little honey to round off the flavor (optional).

Serve squash on individual plates topped with a generous portion of sauce and sprinkled with grated cheese.

1 spaghetti squash

4 tbsp olive oil

1 onion, chopped

2 cloves garlic, chopped

1 carrot, finely cubed

1 leek, sliced

1 rib celery, chopped

1oz/25g dried mushrooms, rehydrated for 15 minutes in warm water and chopped

15oz/400g cooked French green lentils

½ tsp each thyme, oregano and basil

1 bay leaf

2fl oz/¼ cup/60ml red wine

2fl oz/¼ cup/60ml unsweetened almond milk

15oz/400g tomatoes, chopped

2 tbsp tomato paste

acacia honey (optional)

grated Parmesan or pecorino

salt & freshly ground black pepper

Moujadara

4 tbsp olive oil

5 onions, sliced (not too finely) lengthwise

3 cloves garlic, finely chopped

1 level tsp turmeric

1 level tsp cumin

1 level tsp cinnamon

7oz/1 cup/200g brown basmati rice

13fl oz/1⅔ cup/400 ml vegetable stock (to cook the rice)

9oz/1¼ cup/250g dry lentils (green or brown), soaked overnight

13fl oz/1⅔ cup/400 ml water (to cook the lentils)

1 bay leaf

3 tbsp chopped fresh cilantro or parsley

juice of 1 lemon

2 tbsp gomasio (toasted, ground sesame seeds, available at health-food shops)

salt & freshly ground pepper

This hearty all-in-one grain-and-lentil dish hails from the Eastern Mediterranean. The combination of lentils and whole grains provides high-quality proteins that the body can easily assimilate, which is why many plant-based cuisines combine legumes and grains. Traditionally, this dish is made with wheat or spelt bulgur, but we replace these here with brown basmati rice, which is gluten-free and has a lower glycemic index ranking. Quinoa, another gluten-free, high-protein grain, works well too – nice and crunchy! Serves 4.

In a heavy-bottomed pot on medium heat, heat olive oil and cook lightly salted onions garlic for about 25 minutes, covered, stirring occasionally until soft and golden. Add a little water if they get too dry, or remove lid if they're too wet. When they are quite soft, add garlic and spices and cook for another minute, taking care not to burn spices or they will taste bitter. Set aside.

While the onions are cooking, place rice in a pot, cover with vegetable stock and bring to the boil. Cover and simmer on low heat until nearly done (see packet instructions for cooking time).

Put lentils in a separate pot, add bay leaf and water, bring to the boil, cover and simmer on low heat for 5-10 minutes, or until nearly done (keep checking – soaked lentils soften very quickly).

Once lentils and rice are *al dente*, combine and cook together for another 5 minutes or until both are cooked through. Season with salt and pepper.

Briefly reheat the onions. In a large serving bowl, combine lentil-rice mixture with the onions, season with lemon juice, salt and pepper, and toss gently; the consistency should be light and grainy.

Sprinkle with *gomasio* and chopped coriander or parsley and serve immediately.

Mushroom *orzotto*

A specialty from northern Italy, this is prepared like a classic risotto, only using barley (*orzo* in Italian) instead of rice. This substitution affords many advantages, for barley is rich in anti-cancer nutrients such as selenium, lignans and soluble fiber. It also has a lower GI rating than most types of rice. Barley needs to be soaked overnight; this makes it easier to digest and faster to cook. When buying barley, always choose hulled over pot or pearled barley which undergo more processing and are less nutritious. Serves 4.

In a large skillet on medium heat, warm a tablespoon of olive oil and cook garlic, fresh and rehydrated mushrooms and thyme, stirring regularly, until soft (about 10 minutes).

In a heavy-bottomed pot, heat another tablespoon olive oil on medium heat and gently cook the chopped onion, stirring regularly until it is translucent. Add barley and cook for a minute. Now begin adding stock, ladle by ladle, and keep stirring while the barley grains slowly absorb the liquid.

After about 20 minutes of ladling and stirring you should have used up all the stock. The barley grains will have roughly doubled in volume and the mixture will be creamy. Now add cooked mushrooms and a splash of white wine and cook, stirring, for another 2-3 minutes. If the mixture appears too firm or sticky, add a little more stock, wine or water.

Test the grains: they should be soft but slightly chewy. Season with salt, pepper and lemon juice. Stir in the butter and parsley, transfer to a serving dish and sprinkle with grated cheese.

Variations
- For added protein, add cubed, firm tofu or leftover chicken.
- For a splash of color, stir in some baby spinach leaves, arugula or other fast-wilting greens a minute or two before serving.

---

2 tbsp olive oil

4 cloves garlic, finely chopped

1.1lb/500g mushrooms (e.g. button, chestnut, oyster, shiitake), sliced

1oz/25g dried mushrooms, rehydrated in warm water for 15 minutes

½ tsp thyme

1 onion, finely chopped

7oz/1 cup/200g hulled barley, soaked for 12 hours and drained

1⅔ pints/3½ cups/800ml vegetable or chicken stock

2-3 tbsp dry white wine

squeeze of lemon juice

1 tbsp butter

2 tbsp chopped parsley

grated Parmesan or pecorino cheese

salt & freshly ground black pepper

Vegetables

One of the things I enjoy most about teaching people to cook is helping my students learn to like vegetables. As discussed in Chapter 4, vegetables are an unbeatable source of goodness and people who do not eat them are depriving themselves of the fundamental building blocks of health.

Alas, as children many of us got to know vegetables as khaki-colored, slimy lumps that our parents insisted we eat. Slathered in floury cheese sauces we could just about get them down, but on their own they seemed pretty repugnant.

What I want to do here is to re-acquaint you with vegetables – and this time it's going to be fun! Rather than serving them steamed (big yawn) or boiled (big yuck), we turn them into tangy stews, flavorful mashes, melting *gratins* and even make-believe couscous grains!

My favorite cooking method for vegetables is to braise or steam them in their own juice at moderate temperature. This allows them to soften gently without killing off the vitamins and lets the flavors mingle nicely. Oven-baking is another method I favor when I'm not in a rush; it yields meltingly tender vegetables with a hint of sweetness.

Often I don't use specific vegetable recipes. I simply sweat an onion and some garlic in a little olive oil with a pinch of salt and then add whatever seasonal vegetables my refrigerator holds: peas, beans, asparagus, leeks, mushrooms, bell peppers, carrots, celery, zucchini – sometimes on their own, other times in combination. I add a little water, cover the pan and let it all simmer gently for 10 minutes or so until the vegetables are soft. A drizzle of lemon juice and olive oil, a sprinkling of chopped parsley and it's ready!

Some health-food proponents recommend stir-frying vegetables in a wok, but I am not overly keen on this method: high-temperature cooking of this sort can result in vegetables that are undercooked at the core but overcooked or even burnt on the outside. It's also quite a hectic style of cooking, requiring constant stirring and precise timings. (Moreover, studies have shown that high-temperature wok-cooking can produce carcinogenic fumes.)

So just take your time and enjoy your greens (and reds, and yellows, and oranges, and purples, and pinks ...).

Sicilian eggplant stew

One of Sicily's best-known dishes is *caponata*, a delicious sweet-and-sour stew of meltingly soft eggplants, crunchy celery and pine nuts brought together by fruity tomatoes and rounded off with fragrant basil. Serves 4 as a side dish or *hors d'oeuvre*.

In a dry pan on low heat, toast pine nuts until golden and fragrant (2-3 minutes). Transfer to a plate and set aside.

In a large, heavy-bottomed skillet, heat 2 tablespoons olive oil and cook onion and celery for 5 minutes, stirring regularly until translucent. Add eggplant cubes and remaining olive oil and continue cooking until the eggplant starts to turn golden (about 10 minutes), turning the vegetables occasionally with a spatula to prevent them sticking to the pan.

Add tomatoes, olives, vinegar, capers and honey and cover, simmering on a low heat for another 15 minutes. Just before serving, season to taste with salt and pepper, then sprinkle with basil and pine nuts.

This can be enjoyed warm or cold, on its own or accompanied by eggs, fish, lean meat or plain steamed bulgur or brown rice.

2 tbsp pine nuts

5 tbsp olive oil

1 onion, quartered and sliced

1 rib celery, finely sliced

2 eggplants, diced

15oz/400g tomatoes, chopped

12 black olives, sliced

2 tbsp red wine vinegar

2 tbsp capers

1 tbsp acacia honey

2 tbsp chopped basil or parsley

salt & freshly ground black pepper

Roast asparagus

5 tbsp olive oil

1 clove garlic, crushed

1.1lb/500g asparagus
(green or white)

1 tbsp balsamic vinegar

salt & freshly ground black
pepper

a piece of Parmesan
or pecorino cheese for
shavings

Asparagus, the herald of spring, is a particularly festive vegetable, its elegant green or white spears, crunchy texture and delicate aroma providing a special treat. Try to buy locally grown asparagus – it has much more flavor than its well-travelled cousins from distant shores. Roasting asparagus concentrates its flavor (which, sadly, often gets lost in the cooking water when boiled) while retaining its crunch. Serves 4 as a side dish or *hors d'oeuvre.*

Preheat oven to 350°F/180°C.

In a small bowl, combine olive oil and garlic with a whisk.

Cut any dry or stringy ends off the asparagus. Lay asparagus spears in an ovenproof dish in a single layer, drizzle with garlicky olive oil mixture and toss lightly so the spears are well-coated.

Place in oven and bake for 10-12 minutes, depending on the spears' thickness. Prick the asparagus with a skewer about 2 inches/5cm from the bottom of the stem to test for doneness. When they're easily pierced, they're ready.

Remove the dish from the oven and drizzle asparagus with balsamic vinegar. Shake the dish gently sideways to spread the vinegar, then season with pepper and a little salt. Slice off thin shavings of Parmesan or pecorino with a cheese slicer or kitchen knife and scatter these over the asparagus.

Swiss chard *au gratin*

Instead of the more traditional thick, white *béchamel* sauce I like to use herby tomato sauce to make this nourishing gratin. The tangy tomato flavor masks chard's slightly earthy taste that some people dislike. This recipe works well with spinach too. Serves 4 as a side dish.

Preheat oven to 350°F/180°C. Bring a large pot of water to the boil.

Soak and rinse chard thoroughly in a sink of water (if it's very gritty, use several changes of water). Drain and chop coarsely. When the water is boiling, blanch chard for 1 minute; drain in a strainer. Squeeze out excess moisture by pushing a small bowl onto the greens in the strainer.

Heat tomato sauce in a pot. Add drained chard and mix well. Tip chard-tomato mix into an ovenproof dish and scatter with grated cheese. Bake in the oven for 20 minutes until the cheese is melted and golden.

1⅔ lb/750g fresh Swiss chard, stalks removed

12fl oz/1½ cups/350ml Basic tomato sauce (p. 226)

3.5oz/100g ewes' milk cheese, grated

Braised fennel and onion

This sweet, melting vegetable dish goes particularly well with fish. Serves 4 as a side dish.

In a large, heavy bottomed skillet cook lightly salted onion and garlic in olive oil until translucent. Add fennel slices and cook for 10 minutes, turning occasionally with a spatula. Add wine, cover, reduce heat to lowest setting and stew gently for 10 minutes.

Season with salt, pepper and lemon juice, sprinkle with chopped fennel fronds and serve.

3 bulbs fennel, cored and thinly sliced; save green fronds for garnish

1 large onion, sliced

2 cloves garlic, chopped

2 tbsp olive oil

2fl oz/60ml white wine

salt & black pepper

squeeze of lemon juice

Three ways with Brussels sprouts

It may come as a surprise that Brussels sprouts actually require very little cooking; treated with a light touch, they will reward you with a crunchy texture and unexpected sweetness. The secret behind crisp, sweet Brussels sprouts is to buy them young and fresh, and to minimize cooking time by cutting them into quarters or shredding them finely and removing their tough outer leaves. Each recipe serves 4 as a side dish.

Brussels sprouts & carrots with lemon-mustard dressing

1.1lb/500g Brussels sprouts

1 tbsp olive oil

1 onion, chopped

1-2 cloves garlic, chopped

3 carrots, thinly sliced

2fl oz/¼ cup/60ml stock

1 tbsp parsley, chopped

Lemon-mustard dressing

3 tbsp olive oil

1 tbsp Dijon mustard

1 clove garlic, crushed

pinch of lemon zest (untreated)

juice of ½ lemon

1 tsp acacia honey

salt & black pepper

Start by trimming the sprouts' stems and removing any discolored or wilted outer leaves. Halve sprouts from top to bottom and then cut again into quarters.

Prepare dressing: in a small bowl, combine olive oil, mustard, crushed garlic, lemon juice and zest, salt, pepper and acacia honey and whisk to obtain a smooth emulsion.

In a deep skillet on medium heat, warm olive oil and cook onion and garlic until translucent. Add carrots and stock or water and cook for 6-8 minutes. Add sprouts, cover and cook until vegetables are tender (about 6-8 minutes more). If they get too dry, add a little water.

Remove from heat, drizzle with lemon-mustard dressing, toss lightly, season to taste with salt and pepper, sprinkle with chopped parsley and serve immediately.

Oven-roasted Brussels sprouts

Preheat oven to 350°F/180°C.

Start by trimming the sprouts' stems and removing discolored or wilted outer leaves. Halve sprouts from top to bottom.

In a small bowl, combine olive oil and crushed garlic and whisk. Place sprouts in roasting pan, drizzle with oil-and-garlic emulsion and toss until the sprouts are coated. Slide into the preheated oven. After 10 minutes, stir vegetables and return to oven for another 10 minutes until tender. Remove and season with salt, pepper and lemon juice and serve immediately.

1.1lb/500g Brussels sprouts

3 tbsp olive oil

2 cloves garlic, crushed

salt & black pepper

squeeze of lemon juice

Speedy Mediterranean sprouts

Start by trimming the sprouts' stems and removing discolored or wilted outer leaves. Halve sprouts from top to bottom and cut again into quarters.

In a large skillet, cook onion and garlic in olive oil on medium heat until they are translucent. Add Brussels sprouts and sundried tomatoes and stir gently with a spatula. Add water or stock and cover; cook for about 10 minutes, gently stirring halfway through. Add more water if necessary.

While sprouts are cooking, toast pine nuts in a dry skillet on medium heat for 2-3 minutes until they start to give off a baked fragrance. Transfer to a bowl to cool.

Test sprouts; they should be tender but *al dente* and bright green. Season to taste with salt, pepper and lemon juice. Transfer to serving bowl and scatter with chopped parsley and pine nuts.

2 tbsp olive oil

1 onion, sliced

3 cloves garlic, chopped

1.1lb/500g Brussels sprouts

2oz/50g sundried tomatoes, chopped

2fl oz/60 ml water or stock

2 tbsp pine nuts

2 tbsp parsley, chopped

squeeze of lemon juice

salt & black pepper

Mushrooms *Bordelaise*

2 tbsp olive oil

3 cloves garlic, chopped

15oz/400g mushrooms
(porcini, oyster, chestnut
or other)

squeeze of lemon juice

1 tbsp parsley, finely
chopped

salt & freshly ground
black pepper

This aromatic side dish is quick and easy to prepare. Make a double batch so you can use leftovers for a mushroom omelet (p. 160) or Mushroom soup (p. 146) the next day. Made with porcini mushrooms, this dish tastes dark and earthy; oyster mushrooms lend it a lighter, more summery note. Serves 4 as a side dish.

Clean mushrooms by wiping grit off them with a damp cloth and cutting away any damaged parts. Cut mushrooms (including stalks) into roughly 1-inch/2cm cubes. If using frozen mushrooms, place them in a strainer to defrost and drain.

In a large, heavy-bottomed skillet on medium heat cook garlic for 30 seconds in olive oil. Add mushrooms and cook, stirring regularly, for 10-15 minutes until mushrooms are soft but not soggy; most of their moisture should have evaporated. Sprinkle with parsley and lemon juice, season with salt and pepper.

Broccoli-cauliflower medley

Brighten up winter meals with this quick, simple side dish that makes a welcome change from plain steamed broccoli. Serves 4 as a side dish.

Steam broccoli and cauliflower florets for 5 minutes; tip into a strainer and set aside.

Meanwhile, heat olive oil in a large skillet and cook lightly salted onions and garlic on medium heat for 15 minutes, stirring regularly. When the onions are quite soft, add turmeric and cook for another minute, stirring gently.

Tip steamed broccoli and cauliflower florets into the pan with the onions and cook together for 5 minutes, stirring well to ensure they acquire turmeric's golden glow. Season to taste with salt, pepper and lemon juice and add chopped parsley.

1 head broccoli, cut into florets
1 small cauliflower, cut into florets
3 tbsp olive oil
2 red onions, sliced
3 cloves garlic, chopped
1 tsp turmeric
squeeze of lemon juice
2 tbsp chopped parsley
salt & black pepper

Cauliflower "couscous"

Here's another substitutionist's conjuring trick: replacing a relatively glycemic grain with that low-glycemic anti-cancer favorite: cauliflower! Serves 4 as a side dish.

In a large pot, gently warm olive oil on medium heat and cook chopped onion and garlic until translucent. Add turmeric and cook for another minute, stirring constantly.

In a food processor, chop raw cauliflower until it resembles large bread crumbs. Add cauliflower and 2fl oz/¼ cup/60ml of water to the onions and garlic, cover and cook, stirring regularly, until the cauliflower is *al dente* – about 10 minutes. Season to taste with salt, pepper and a squeeze of lemon juice and serve immediately.

2 tbsp olive oil
1 onion, chopped
2 cloves garlic, chopped
1 tsp turmeric
1 cauliflower, cut into florets
squeeze of lemon
1 tbsp chopped parsley
salt & black pepper

Eggplant "pizzas"

2 large, firm eggplants

2fl oz/¼ cup/60ml olive oil

7fl oz/scant 1 cup/200ml Basic tomato sauce (p. 226)

6oz/170g roast peppers in olive oil (home-made (p. 120) or from a jar)

15 sliced chestnut or button mushrooms

3oz/85g feta or mozzarella cheese

10 black olives, chopped or sliced

4 tbsp pine nuts

These are very easy to make, and quick, too, if you have Basic tomato sauce (p. 226) in your refrigerator or freezer. If you haven't and are in a hurry, store-bought pesto or tomato paste work fine. The eggplant acts as the "pizza crust" onto which you can pile any number of vegetables, nuts, fish (e.g., anchovies, tinned mackerel or sardines), seeds, olives, capers, cheeses, etc. The version below contains seven vegetables (including those used to make the sauce)! Serves 4 as a side dish or *hors d'oeuvre*.

Preheat grill to medium.

With a long knife, cut off a thin slice on either side of the eggplants, and then slice the rest of the eggplants into 4-5 slices approximately as thick as your index finger.

Cover a baking tray with parchment and lay eggplant slices on it; lightly brush both sides with olive oil and slide under the grill. Grill 5-6 minutes on each side until golden.

Remove and spread tomato sauce onto each eggplant slice. Top with grilled peppers, mushrooms, cheese, olives and pine nuts or anything else you would top a pizza with. Grill for another 8-10 minutes until the toppings begin to turn golden and the cheese has melted.

Lift onto plates with a spatula. To really boost your vegetable quota, serve with a mixed salad or steamed vegetables of your choice.

Variation

These taste delicious on slices of sourdough bread that have been lightly toasted, rubbed with fresh garlic and drizzled with olive oil, Spanish *tapa*-style.

Leeks *Provençal*

This dish is inspired by the garlicky vegetable salads widely eaten in the south of France. Here we use leeks, an affordable and delicious vegetable that's available year-round, but you can apply this treatment to a wide range of other vegetables, such as asparagus, green beans, carrots or braised celery. Serves 4 as an hors d'oeuvre or light main meal, served with a slice of crusty bread.

Clean leeks: cut off rootlets, discard outer layer and remove about 6-8 inches/15-20cm of the dark green ends. With a sharp knife, slice lengthwise down the outermost 2-3 layers of each leek, fold back the leaves and rinse thoroughly under running water to remove any remaining grit. If the leeks are very fat, slice in half lengthwise.

Cut leeks into roughly 8-inch/20-cm lengths and steam for 15-20 minutes (depending on thickness) until tender but still a light, fresh shade of green. (Prick with a kitchen knife of fork – it should slide easily into the leeks when they're fully cooked.) Remove from steamer with kitchen tongs and place in a high-rimmed serving dish.

While the leeks are cooking, prepare the dressing: combine oil, vinegar, garlic, mustard, honey, lemon zest, salt and pepper in a small bowl or blender and whisk into a thick emulsion. Drizzle over the leeks and shake the serving dish to spread the dressing around.

Scatter with chopped anchovies, egg, parsley and olives. This dish can be enjoyed warm or chilled for a few hours (when the flavors have had time to infuse).

1.5lb/700g firm, slender leeks

3 hard-boiled eggs, cooled, peeled & chopped

3 anchovy fillets in olive oil, drained and finely chopped

1 tbsp anchovies in olive oil, drained and finely chopped

2 tbsp parsley, chopped

1¾ oz/¼ cup/50g black olives, pitted and coarsely chopped

Dressing

3.5fl oz/scant ½ cup/100ml olive oil

2 tbsp red wine vinegar

1 clove garlic, crushed

1 tbsp mustard (Dijon style)

1 tsp acacia honey

pinch (untreated) grated lemon zest

salt & freshly ground black pepper

Ruby melt

4 tbsp olive oil

3 onions, cut lengthwise into eighths

3 cloves garlic, sliced

4 carrots, peeled and sliced diagonally

2 cooked beets, halved and sliced

juice of ½ lemon

1 tbsp chopped parsley

salt & black pepper

This dish delivers what its name promises: a pile of luscious, deep-red root vegetables that simply melt in your mouth. The natural sweetness of root vegetables and onions braised slowly in their own juice contrasts nicely with the sharp tang of lemon. Serves 4 as a side dish.

In a heavy-bottomed pot, gently warm olive oil on medium heat. Add onions, garlic and carrots and salt lightly. Reduce heat to lowest setting, cover and braise vegetables gently for 15 minutes until they begin to soften; if they stick to the pan, add a little water.

Add beets and continue cooking until the onions are wilted and the carrots soft (about 10 minutes). Season with lemon juice, salt and pepper, sprinkle with parsley and serve.

Cauliflower mash

3 tbsp olive oil

1 onion, chopped

2 cloves garlic, chopped

2 leeks, sliced

1 tsp turmeric

1 cauliflower, coarsely chopped

3.5fl oz/scant ½ cup/100ml stock or water

squeeze of lemon juice

2 tbsp chopped parsley

salt & black pepper

If you are fond of mashed potato but are trying to cut back on that glycemic tuber, this fragrant golden mash is for you. A delicious accompaniment to any "saucy" dish. Serves 4 as a side dish.

In a heavy-bottomed pot, heat 1 tablespoon olive oil and add onion, garlic and leeks, salt lightly and cook for 5 minutes. Add turmeric and pepper and cook another minute, stirring.

Add cauliflower and stir well so the yellow color of the turmeric coats the cauliflower evenly. Add stock or water, cover and cook for 10-12 minutes or until the cauliflower is soft.

With a hand-held blender, puree vegetables to the desired consistency. Season with salt, pepper and lemon juice. Drizzle with the remaining olive oil, sprinkle with chopped parsley and serve.

Creamy leek and carrot *compote*

Compote in French denotes a dessert of stewed fruit; however, *compoter* also describes the process by which food – sweet or savory – is gently cooked using very little water so that the ingredients are reduced to a soft, melting stew with the nutrients preserved by the low heat while the flavors have had time to blend. Serves 4 as a side dish.

In a heavy-bottomed skillet on medium heat, gently warm olive oil and add leeks, garlic and carrots and turmeric, white wine or water and sprinkle with salt. Once the vegetables start to bubble gently, cover and reduce heat to lowest setting. Stew gently for 20 minutes, stirring occasionally. Add a little water if the mixture seems too dry.

When the vegetables are soft, stir in lemon juice and Cashew cream. Sprinkle with chopped parsley and serve.

Variation

For a more exotic flavor, replace Cashew cream with coconut cream added just before serving and sprinkle with chopped cilantro.

2 tbsp olive oil

4-5 leeks, finely sliced

2 cloves garlic, chopped

4-5 carrots, sliced

1 level tsp turmeric

4 tbsp white wine or water

squeeze of lemon juice

3 tbsp Cashew cream (p. 231)

2 tbsp chopped parsley

salt & freshly ground black pepper

Garlicky spinach

1.5lb/700g fresh leaf
spinach

2 tbsp olive oil

5 cloves garlic, finely sliced

pinch of nutmeg

squeeze of lemon juice

salt & freshly ground black
pepper

I don't usually boil vegetables in water but make an exception here as this removes the tart bitterness caused by the oxalic acid in spinach that puts so many people off this delicious vegetable. Serves 4 as a side dish.

Bring a large pot of water to the boil.

Thoroughly wash spinach in water (several changes of water if very gritty) and remove hard stems. Drain in a strainer and chop coarsely.

When the water boils, throw in the spinach and cook for 1 minute; any longer and the spinach will lose its flavor and beautiful green color. Drain in the strainer, squeezing out excess moisture.

Warm 1 tablespoon olive oil in a heavy-bottomed pan on medium heat. Add the finely sliced garlic and sauté for 30 seconds. Tip the drained spinach into the garlicky oil and reheat, gently mixing spinach and oil. Add the second tablespoon of oil, season with salt, pepper, nutmeg and lemon juice, toss lightly and serve.

If you can't find fresh spinach, frozen spinach is nearly as tasty; however, as it is blanched before freezing, skip the boiling stage. Simply add defrosted spinach to the garlic in the pan and cook on low heat until warmed through; season to taste.

Variations
- For a creamier dish, stir in a little Cashew cream (p. 231) or *crème fraiche.*
- A pinch of lemon zest instead of nutmeg adds summery freshness.

Pumpkin mash

Pumpkin and squash are not only simple to prepare and highly versatile, they also taste sweet and starchy (with a moderate glycemic index ranking, see pp. 42-43) and add a beautiful shot of color to your plate. Most importantly, they provide a bounty of nutrients, including antioxidant carotenoids.

My favorite is Hokkaido squash, whose tender, edible skin makes it a boon for the lazy or time-starved cook. Butternut squash works well too here, and can be easily peeled with a potato peeler. For a more exotic flavor, add 1 teaspoon grated fresh ginger and sprinkle with chopped cilantro leaves. Serves 4 as a side dish.

Clean the squash thoroughly on the outside, using a soft brush under running water. Remove stem and halve squash with a long, heavy knife. Scoop out the seeds.

Chop squash into 1-inch/2-cm cubes (the smaller the cubes, the faster they cook and the fewer nutrients will be destroyed) and place in a large, heavy-bottomed pot.

Add water, cover and bring to the boil. Once boiling, reduce heat and simmer until squash is soft (about 15 minutes). With a hand-held electric blender, mash the squash with its cooking water until you have a smooth, creamy puree.

Add garlic and olive oil and stir well. Sprinkle with chopped parsley and serve immediately.

1 Hokkaido squash

10fl oz/1¼ cups/300ml water

2 cloves garlic, finely chopped

2 tbsp olive oil

2 tbsp parsley, chopped

salt & freshly ground black pepper

Oven-roasted *ratatouille*

2 bell peppers (red, yellow or green)

1 large onion, chopped

4 cloves garlic, finely chopped

1 eggplant, cubed (½-to-1-inch/1-to-2-cm cubes)

2 zucchini, cubed (½-to-1-inch/1-to-2-cm cubes)

3 tomatoes, coarsely chopped

1 tsp thyme

½ tsp each of ground coriander and finely chopped rosemary

3 tbsp olive oil + 1 tbsp for drizzling

1-2 tbsp chopped parsley or fresh cilantro

squeeze of lemon juice

salt & freshly ground black pepper

Nothing could be simpler than this tasty southern French summer vegetable dish. All you need to do is a bit of chopping and then let your oven take care of the rest. *Ratatouille* tastes great as a side dish with fish or meat, cold as a salad or as a filling for omelets. It also freezes well, so why not make a double batch and save some for another time? You can adapt the vegetable ratios to your liking – these are just rough guidelines. Serves 4 as a side dish.

Preheat oven to 400°F/200°C.

Place all the chopped vegetables in a large ovenproof dish. Drizzle with oil, scatter with thyme, ground coriander and rosemary and toss carefully so all the vegetables are coated.

Slide into the oven and roast, turning with a spatula every 10 minutes to ensure even cooking and to avoid the top layer getting burnt. The vegetables should be ready after about 30 minutes.

Drizzle with the remaining olive oil, season with salt, pepper and lemon juice, scatter with chopped herbs and serve.

Spiced red cabbage with apples

This wintery comfort dish goes perfectly with roast duck, goose or any other poultry. It gets better after a day or two, so if you can cook it in advance, so much the better.

Remove outer cabbage leaves and discard. Quarter cabbage, remove core and slice into thin strips.

In a heavy-bottomed pot on medium heat, gently warm oil and cook onion until translucent. Add apples and cook for another 3 minutes. Add sliced cabbage and continue cooking while stirring constantly.

Now add vinegar, red wine, bay leaf, spices and honey and combine. Add water or apple juice, whichever using, cover tightly and simmer on low heat.

Stir several times and make sure there's enough moisture in the pot so the cabbage doesn't stick. Keep testing for done-ness: young, tender cabbage is ready after 30 minutes. Season with salt and black pepper.

1 medium red cabbage
2 tbsp olive oil
1 onion, coarsely chopped
2 apples, cubed
2 tbsp red wine vinegar
4 tbsp red wine
1 cinnamon stick, 1 pinch ground ginger, 1 pinch ground coriander, 1 clove, 1 cardamom pod
1-2 tbsp acacia honey
1 bay leaf
9fl oz/1 cup/250ml water or apple juice
salt & black pepper

Marinades, sauces, dressings, creams

Just like a stylish fashion accessory can smarten up a modest outfit, intensely flavored sauces, dressings and marinades can spruce up the most humble dish. They should never overpower food but should complement it in such a way that its own essential flavors are enhanced. Meanwhile, with foods that have little flavor of their own – such as tofu or chicken breast – they can add much-needed gustatory interest.

Flavor-packed culinary accessories are also great time- and money-savers. Take, for example, a jar of pesto, that wonderful refrigerator stand-by. You can stir a teaspoonful into omelet batter, spread another on toast and top it with tinned sardines, marinate tofu in it overnight or use it to jazz up plain tomato sauce. Smear it onto fish or chicken before baking these in the oven, or simply stir it into hot pasta. Because it is so intensely flavored and keeps well in the refrigerator, it's economical, too.

Other time-savers we explore in the following section are bottled salad dressings that you can make in advance and store in the refrigerator.

How often have you thought: "I'd like to eat a salad tonight, but I just don't have the energy to make a dressing…"? With a bottle of home-made dressing to hand (which takes the same amount of time to prepare as a single batch of dressing) all you need to do is throw some salad greens into a bowl and drizzle with your dressing (which will be a great deal healthier, tastier and more economical than a pre-made commercial dressing).

Several of the recipes in the next section offer a useful way of getting anti-cancer foods we don't often eat – especially herbs and spices – into our diet in small but regular doses. Thus the home-made ketchup (rich in lycopene, garlic, onions and spices), turmeric chutney (turmeric, ginger, onions, cinnamon, lemon zest) or the three aromatic pestos that follow are packed with health-protective ingredients but don't taste even remotely medicinal.

For let's remember that healthy food shouldn't only be "good for you." In order to attain its full health-enhancing potential, food should be enjoyable – something you look forward to eating day after day!

Homemade tomato ketchup

If you think making your own ketchup is a little over-the-top, consider the advantages. Not only are you avoiding the drawbacks of mass-produced ketchup – excess sugar, salt and various additives. In addition, this ketchup enables you to consume small but regular doses of anti-cancer spices and foods throughout the day! Enjoy a small blob with your breakfast egg, another on your lunchbox sandwich and a third with fish or chicken for dinner – among countless other options. Makes about 2 pints/1l.

In a medium-sized pot on medium heat, gently cook the onion in olive oil until translucent. Add spices and cook for another minute, stirring continually.

Now add tomatoes, tomato paste, apricots, vinegar, salt and pepper. Bring to the boil, then reduce heat and cook for 30 minutes on the lowest setting. If using tomatoes from a jar, cover with a lid. If using fresh tomatoes (these generally contain more water), leave uncovered so that excess moisture can evaporate.

Transfer to a blender and liquidize to obtain a smooth, thick puree. If it is too thick, add a little water or apple juice. For an extra-smooth sauce, pass through a sieve. Season with a little more salt, vinegar and honey if necessary.

Fill into an empty, thoroughly cleaned glass bottle. Well-sealed, this keeps in the refrigerator for at least two weeks.

2 tbsp olive oil

1 onion, chopped

½ tsp gingerbread spice (or a generous pinch each of ginger, cloves, cinnamon and nutmeg)

1 tsp turmeric

1¾lb/800g tomatoes, chopped

3 tbsp tomato paste

3.5oz/⅔ cup/100g dried apricots, chopped

2 tbsp apple cider vinegar

1 tbsp acacia honey (optional)

salt & freshly ground black pepper

Three tomato sauces

Ready-made tomato sauces usually contain unhealthy oils, too much sugar and salt and often have a rather conserved flavor. Since they're so easy to prepare from scratch and are wonderful vehicles for anti-cancer ingredients such as tomatoes, onions, garlic, olive oil and herbs, I recommend that you make large batches of tomato sauce and freeze these. This way, when you come home after a tiring day, all you need to do is whip a portion of sauce out of refrigerator or freezer, reheat and enjoy! Each recipe yields about 2 pints/800ml of sauce.

Basic tomato sauce

2 tbsp olive oil

2 onions, chopped

2 cloves garlic, chopped

1¾lb/800g tomatoes, coarsely chopped

½ tsp each of thyme and oregano

1 bay leaf

3 tbsp tomato paste

salt & freshly ground black pepper

acacia honey (optional)

This can be made in 15 minutes if you're in a hurry, but the longer you let it simmer, the better it will taste. Unseasoned, unsalted tomatoes in jars are fine if you can't get fresh ones.

In a heavy-bottomed pot, gently warm olive oil and cook onion and garlic until translucent. Add tomatoes, herbs and tomato paste, bring to the boil, cover and simmer on low heat for at least 15 minutes. If it seems too thick, add some water or a splash of white or red wine.

Remove bay leaf. Transfer sauce to blender and liquidize until smooth and creamy. Season with salt and pepper; add a little acacia honey if it is too acidic.

Raw tomato sauce

This fresh-off-the-vine sauce is best in the summer when tomatoes are bursting with flavor. Alas, it doesn't freeze well, so enjoy straight away. Delicious served over hot pasta, cooked navy beans or lightly steamed vegetables.

Coarsely chop the tomatoes and place in a blender with the olive oil. Squeeze the garlic into the blender jug with a garlic press and add the herbs and tomato paste. Liquidize on top speed for about 30 seconds or until you obtain a thick, smooth emulsion. Season with salt and pepper. If the sauce is too acidic, add a touch of acacia honey.

2.2lb/1kg sun-ripened tomatoes

2fl oz/¼ cup/60ml olive oil

2 cloves garlic, crushed

3-4 tbsp fresh basil leaves

1 tsp fresh oregano leaves

2 tbsp tomato paste

salt & black pepper

V7 tomato sauce

This is a great way of sneaking vegetables onto a veggiephobe's plate: as the tomato taste dominates, the eater will have no idea the sauce contains seven vegetables – each and every one an anti-cancer ingredient!

In a large, heavy-bottomed pot, gently warm the olive oil and cook onion and garlic until translucent. Add carrots, leek, celery, add 2 tablespoons water, cover and cook on low heat for 10 minutes, stirring occasionally.

When the leeks and carrots are soft, add mushrooms, herbs and chopped tomatoes and bring to the boil. Cover and simmer on low heat for 30 minutes, or longer if you have time. If the sauce is too thick, add a little water or a splash of wine.

When the vegetables are soft, remove bay leaves, transfer to a blender and liquidize until the sauce is smooth and creamy. Season to taste with salt and pepper, adding a little acacia honey if the sauce is too acidic.

2 tbsp olive oil

1 onion, coarsely chopped

2 cloves garlic, chopped

2 carrots, cubed

1 leek, finely sliced

1 rib celery, cubed

7oz/2 cups/200g fresh mushrooms, chopped

2 bay leaves

½ tsp each thyme, oregano and basil

1¾ lb/800g tomatoes

salt & black pepper

Three ways with pesto

All along the shores of the Mediterranean, cooks have traditionally pounded together oils, spices and pungent herbs to make aromatic pastes that can be mixed into almost everything. Because these preparations were usually prepared in a pestle and mortar, they are called "pesto." I confess I don't usually use a pestle and mortar, preferring electric food processors for speed and ease of preparation. Here are my three favorite pesto-style sauces.

Moroccan *chermoula*

6-8 heaped tbsp cilantro leaves

3 tbsp parsley leaves

3 tbsp olive oil

2 cloves garlic, chopped

2 tbsp paprika powder

1 tsp ground cumin

1 tsp ground coriander

1 tsp turmeric

1 tsp salt

1 tsp finely grated fresh ginger

juice of ½ lemon

pinch of grated lemon zest (untreated)

pinch of chili powder (optional)

large pinch of saffron, soaked in 1 tbsp warm water for 10 minutes

North African *chermoula* is a delicious herbal emulsion made of fresh herbs, oil, cilantro, cumin, lemon and paprika. It goes beautifully with most vegetables, oily fish (whose pungent flavors it matches well) or chicken and can also be used to marinate these. Makes 8-10 tablespoons.

Combine all the ingredients in a small electric food processor and blend into a smooth paste. Store in a tightly sealed container. This keeps in the refrigerator for at least a week.

Walnut *tarator*

Tarator, a delicious garlicky walnut paste, hails from Lebanon and Turkey. In some regions, it is prepared as a refreshing cold soup that also includes cucumbers and yogurt. The thicker version here can be enjoyed as a topping for cooked or grilled vegetables, with fish or poultry, spooned onto hot pasta or as a dip for raw vegetables. Makes 8-10 tablespoons.

Place nuts, garlic, oil and lemon juice in a small blender and blend until they form a creamy emulsion. Add water to obtain the desired consistency. Stir in dill or parsley and season with salt and pepper. Chilled in a tightly sealed container this keeps for at least a week.

3.5oz/scant 1 cup/100g walnuts (or half walnuts, half pine nuts)

1 large clove garlic, crushed

4 tbsp olive oil

2 tbsp lemon juice

a few tbsp water

1 tsp dill or parsley, chopped

salt & black pepper

Classic basil pesto

The most famous pesto is Italy's *pesto alla Genovese* which combines fresh basil leaves, pine nuts, Parmesan, garlic and olive oil. In southern France, pine nuts and cheese are omitted (See *Pistou*, p. 149). For a spicier version, replace half the basil with arugula leaves. So-called "winter pesto" can be made by replacing basil with flat-leaf parsley. Makes 8-10 tablespoons.

Place all the ingredients except for the cheese in a food processor and blend into a smooth paste. Transfer to a small mixing bowl. Stir in the cheese and season to taste with pepper and lemon juice; chill. In a tightly sealed container, this keeps for at least a week.

2oz/50g fresh basil leaves

2 cloves garlic, crushed

2oz/50g pine nuts

3oz/¹⁄₃ cup/80ml olive oil

2oz/50g freshly grated Parmesan or pecorino cheese

salt & black pepper

squeeze of lemon juice

Turmeric chutney

2 tbsp olive oil

2 onions, chopped

3 cloves garlic, chopped

1 tsp freshly grated ginger

2 tsp ground turmeric

1 tsp paprika

1 cinnamon stick

3 apples, cored and chopped

6 dried apricots, finely chopped

1½ oz/¼ cup/40g raisins

grated zest of ½ lemon (untreated)

juice of 1 lemon

juice of 1 orange

1-2 tbsp acacia honey (optional)

2 tbsp walnuts, chopped

salt & freshly ground black pepper

This condiment is a tasty way of regularly consuming turmeric, a spice that doesn't always sit easily with western palates. It's also packed with other cancer-protective foods including apples, lemon juice and zest, raisins, apricots, garlic, onions, ginger and cinnamon. A delicious accompaniment to fish, meat, tofu and eggs and sure to liven up any sandwich. Presented in an attractive jar, this makes a great gift for health-conscious people. Makes about two 15oz/400g jars.

In a heavy-bottomed pot on medium heat, warm olive oil and gently cook onions, garlic, ginger and turmeric until the onions are translucent.

Add paprika, cinnamon stick, apples, apricots, raisins, lemon zest, lemon and orange juice, salt and pepper and cover; cook on lowest heat for 30 minutes, stirring occasionally. Add a splash of water if the mixture looks dry or sticks to the pot.

When all the ingredients are soft, remove cinnamon stick and puree chutney to the desired consistency with a hand-held blender. If you prefer chunky chutney, leave whole. (I like mine semi-pureed – just a few chunks amid a fairly smooth puree.)

Season with salt, pepper, lemon juice and honey (if using). Add chopped walnuts and transfer to a tightly sealed jar or container. Well sealed, this keeps in the refrigerator for at least a week.

Cashew cream

Dairy cream is one of the magic ingredients of French cuisine. Its velvety texture and milky flavor lend many French soups, stews and sauces a satisfying richness. The snag: some people find dairy hard to digest, others seek to avoid the saturated fats in dairy cream.

My solution is Cashew cream. It shares dairy cream's sweet, comforting flavor and can be used in much the same way. It is easy to make at home, and contains healthy monounsaturated fatty acids and a range of important minerals. Cashew nuts keep well in the refrigerator; store them in airtight containers so they do not take on refrigerator smells.

You can enjoy Cashew cream cold – poured over dessert, for example – or use it in cooking. It thickens and binds when heated, thus making it a perfect thickener. It's best to soak cashews overnight as this makes the cream more unctuous and reduces the amount of phytic acid in them, thus optimizing mineral absorption. Makes about 12 fl oz/1 ½ cups/350ml.

9oz/2 ¼ cups/250g unsalted, raw cashew nuts, soaked overnight in water

---

7fl oz/scant 1 cup/200ml water

pinch of salt

Drain soaking water, place nuts and fresh water in a small blender and whizz for about 2 minutes or until you obtain a smooth, velvety cream. Add more water for a thinner consistency. Store in a sealable container in the refrigerator; keeps for up to 3 days.

Spicy Cashew cream
Place cashews, water and salt in the blender and add ½ tsp turmeric, ½ tsp ground ginger, freshly ground black pepper and 1 clove crushed garlic; pulse to combine and add water to thin if necessary. This spicy golden cream can be drizzled over soups, stews, meat or fish.

Lemon Cashew cream
Add the zest of ½ lemon and a squeeze of lemon juice to the basic cashew cream recipe and blend as instructed. For sweet cream served with dessert, add a teaspoon of acacia honey; or leave it out and use the cream in sauces or soups for a hint of lemony freshness.

Vanilla Cashew cream
Delicious with cakes and desserts. Just add 1 tsp natural vanilla extract (or scrape the seeds from ½ pod of vanilla) and 1 tsp acacia honey along with the above ingredients and blend as instructed.

Avocado cream

The delicate light-green color of avocado cream is beautifully offset when drizzled over dark vegetable soups (for instance spinach or beet soup) or pink or white fish. The recipes below also make great dips for raw vegetable sticks.

Avocado aioli

This is inspired by *aioli*, a Provençal garlic mayonnaise that's traditionally served as a dip for lightly steamed, mixed vegetables, hard-boiled eggs and salt cod.

1 ripe avocado

1 tbsp lemon juice

1 clove garlic, crushed

1 tbsp olive oil

salt & freshly ground black pepper

Combine all ingredients in a blender and pulse until creamy, adding cold water one tablespoon at a time to achieve the desired consistency. Chill for an hour before serving.

Herby Avocado cream

A delicious dip for crunchy vegetable sticks or on whole grain crackers. Works well as an accompaniment to grilled, baked or steamed fish or white meat.

1 ripe avocado

2 tbsp plain yogurt

squeeze of lemon juice

salt & freshly ground black pepper

2 tbsp fresh herbs, chopped (any green kitchen herbs such as parsley, chives, cilantro, basil, marjoram, dill or a mix of these)

Blend avocado, yogurt, lemon juice and salt in a hand-held blender, adding water if a thinner consistency is desired. Add chopped herbs and pulse briefly to combine. A crushed clove of garlic will lend extra oomph.

Avocado-Blue cheese cream

This is delicious stirred into Broccoli soup (p. 138) or as a dip for vegetable sticks.

1 ripe avocado

2oz/50g Roquefort or any other blue cheese, crumbled

a few tablespoons cold water

Combine all the ingredients in a blender and pulse into a smooth cream, adding cold water one spoonful at a time until you achieve the desired consistency.

Three marinades

These marinades add flavor and color to chicken, turkey or fish and help to reduce the risks inherent in meat cooking (pp. 49-50). They are all prepared and used in the same way: place ingredients in a blender and pulse into a thin paste. Coat meat or fish with them, marinate for at least an hour (ideally overnight) in the refrigerator and then cook as gently as possible. Don't add salt to the marinade as this dries out the meat; lightly salt the foods just before serving. Each recipe makes about 3.5fl oz/ scant ½ cup/100ml. Fresh marinades keep for 3-4 days in the refrigerator. Do not re-use; discard leftovers.

Lemon and garlic marinade
A summery marinade that works well with chicken, turkey and fresh squid.

4 cloves garlic, roughly chopped

juice of 1 lemon

grated zest of ½ lemon (untreated)

3 tbsp herbs (e.g. oregano, rosemary, parsley, sage)

1 tsp turmeric

6 tbsp olive oil

freshly ground black pepper

Mustard marinade
Perfect for flavoring chicken, turkey or tofu.

4 tbsp mustard (2 grainy, 2 smooth)

2fl oz/¼ cup/60ml olive oil

3 tbsp lemon juice

grated zest of ½ lemon (untreated)

3 cloves garlic, crushed

1 tbsp rosemary, chopped

Spicy barbecue-style marinade
This marinade lends succulent flavors to oven-roast or grilled chicken.

2 tsp fresh ginger, finely grated

2 cloves garlic, crushed

1 tsp turmeric

4 tbsp tomato ketchup (p. 225)

juice of ½ orange

grated zest of ½ orange (untreated)

2 tbsp tamari (wheat-free soy sauce)

2 tbsp honey

freshly ground black pepper

Three dressings

You will eat salads more often if you get into the habit of storing home-made, ready-to-use dressings in the refrigerator. They take just as long to prepare as an individual portion, but a bottle containing 1 pint/500ml will dress about 10 salads! These dressings can also be used to jazz up steamed vegetables such as broccoli, asparagus and green beans. Yield: about 1 pint/500ml.

Turmeric and ginger dressing

Delicious on shredded cabbage sprinkled with toasted sesame seeds and fresh cilantro.

7fl oz/scant 1 cup/200ml canola oil

2fl oz/¼ cup/60ml Chinese rice vinegar

3 tbsp toasted sesame oil

2 tbsp tahini (sesame paste)

2 tbsp acacia honey (more or less to taste)

1 tbsp turmeric

½ tbsp finely grated fresh ginger

salt

Combine ingredients in a blender and pulse into a smooth emulsion. Season with salt and pour into a sealable glass bottle. Keeps at least 2 weeks in the refrigerator. Shake before use.

Classic French vinaigrette

A great all-rounder, matches most salads and raw or cooked vegetables.

10fl oz/1¼ cup/300ml oil (half olive, half walnut, canola or hazelnut)

3.5fl oz/scant ½ cup/100ml red wine vinegar

2 tbsp acacia honey (more or less to taste)

1 tbsp whole grain mustard

pinch of herbes de Provence

salt & freshly ground black pepper

Combine ingredients in a blender and pulse into a smooth emulsion. Season and pour into a sealable glass bottle. Keeps at least 2 weeks in the refrigerator. Shake before use.

Italian dressing

A fruity, summery dressing redolent of Mediterranean aromas.

10fl oz/1¼ cup/300ml olive oil

2fl oz/¼ cup/60ml lemon juice

2 tbsp white wine vinegar

2 tbsp honey (more or less to taste)

1 clove garlic, crushed

2 anchovy fillets, rinsed and mashed (optional)

salt & freshly ground black pepper

Combine ingredients in a blender and pulse into a smooth emulsion. Season and pour into a sealable glass bottle. Keeps at least 2 weeks in the refrigerator. Shake before use.

Savory *coulis*

Coulis (pronounced "coolee") is the French word for concentrated fruit- or vegetable-based sauces that are low in calories but bursting with flavor. They make the perfect accompaniment to meat or fish, egg-based dishes (e.g. the Green soufflé on p. 157) or poured over plain steamed vegetables, drizzled into soups or mixed with freshly cooked legumes. Store in refrigerator for 2-3 days, tightly sealed.

Red pepper and onion coulis

2 tbsp olive oil

1 large onion, sliced

2 cloves garlic, chopped

2 red bell peppers, coarsely chopped

about 2fl oz/¼ cup/60ml water

1 tbsp tomato paste

salt & freshly ground black pepper

In a medium-sized pot, cook onion and garlic in olive oil until translucent. Add peppers, water and tomato paste and cover; cook on low heat for 15 minutes until the peppers are soft. In a blender, or with a hand-held pureeing device, liquidize into a smooth sauce, adding a little water if desired. Season with salt and pepper and serve hot or cold. Delicious with fish, omelet or green vegetables.

Parsley coulis

An intensely green, fragrant sauce that tastes wonderful with white fish or meat. You can replace some of the parsley with cilantro and/or mint for a more complex flavor.

2 bunches flat-leaf parsley

2 spring onions, green parts only

1 clove garlic, coarsely chopped

3.5fl oz/scant ½ cup/100ml water

2 tbsp olive oil

lemon juice

salt & freshly ground black pepper

Boil a large pot of salted water and fill a separate bowl with cold water. When the water is boiling, place parsley, spring onions and garlic into the water and blanch for 60 seconds. Drain in a strainer and transfer to the cold water.

Pat herbs dry, remove the thickest stems of the parsley and place the rest in a food processor. Pulse until you have a smooth puree. Add small amounts of water as you blend the herbs until you obtain the desired consistency.

Add olive oil and season to taste with salt, pepper and lemon juice.

Breakfast

Breakfast in the Mediterranean region has traditionally been a lighter and less elaborate affair than in cooler northern climes. However, modern western breakfast habits everywhere have converged towards nutrient-poor meals featuring white bread, pastries, sugary spreads, processed cereals, glycemic juices and caffeine. This may be a good way to get going in the morning, but it's not effective if you want to *keep* going until lunchtime.

By disrupting our blood-sugar balance, breakfasts rich in refined grains and sugar set us up for fluctuating energy levels and "snack attacks" later in the day. This type of meal is also a missed opportunity: why fill up on empty calories when we could be eating nutrient-packed foods? Let's get in the habit of seeing *every* meal – not just lunch or dinner – as an opportunity to eat high-quality nutrients.

In this section, therefore, I focus less on typically Mediterranean breakfast foods and more on nutrient-rich dishes to nourish our bodies until lunchtime. Among others, they all include some form of protein, which is woefully absent from the starchy breakfasts many people eat. Protein provides a feeling of satiety and helps to stabilize blood-sugar levels; it is therefore important to eat it at every meal, and especially for breakfast.

Protein-rich breakfast foods include eggs, nut butters, bread or muesli made with whole grains, seeds and nuts, yogurt or white cheese. In some cultures, notably in Scandinavia and parts of Asia, people eat fish or meat for breakfast; so why not enjoy sardines, cold chicken breast or beans on wholegrain toast at the start of the day?

In some Mediterranean regions, such as Lebanon, Egypt and Turkey and further east, a typical breakfast might consist of a salad of cucumbers, tomatoes, onions, mint and olive oil, pita bread dipped in *labneh* (a rich type of yogurt) or in olive oil and *za'atar* (a mix of thyme, oregano, marjoram and toasted sesame seeds). *Hummus* (p. 192), *ful medames* (cooked and mashed fava beans served with olive oil, parsley, onion, garlic and lemon juice) and *falafel* (p. 190) are enjoyed on weekends.

Three smoothies

Even the most time-starved person should be able to find the time to whizz up a nourishing smoothie in the morning. Each of these smoothies provides healthy fats, antioxidants, protein, fiber and two servings of fruit; not a single empty calorie in sight! For extra fiber, omega-3 fats and lignans (p. 72) add 1 tablespoon of ground flax seeds to any of these smoothies. Each recipe serves 2.

Berry booster

7oz/1 1/3 cup/200g raspberries or blueberries, fresh or frozen

1 tbsp almond butter

1 ripe banana

5fl oz/2/3 cup/150ml almond or hazelnut milk

7oz/scant 1 cup/200g plain yogurt

1 tbsp chopped almonds

Place all the ingredients except the chopped almonds in a blender and whizz into a velvety cream. Pour into tall glasses and sprinkle with almonds.

Apricot awakening

5fl oz/2/3 cup/150ml Apricot coulis (see p. 261) or 3-4 ripe, soft fresh apricots

1 tbsp almond butter

7oz/scant 1 cup/200 g plain yogurt

5fl oz/2/3 cup/150ml hazelnut or almond milk

2 mint leaves

Place all the ingredients except the mint leaves in a blender and whizz into a velvety cream. Pour into tall glasses and decorate with a mint leaf.

Chocolate-hazelnut delight

9fl oz/1 cup/250 ml hazelnut milk

2 tbsp hazelnut butter

2 tbsp pure cocoa powder

1 ripe banana

1 tbsp acacia honey

7oz/scant 1 cup/200g plain yogurt

1 tbsp coarsely chopped hazelnuts

Place all the ingredients except the chopped hazelnuts in a blender and whizz into a velvety cream. Pour into tall glasses and sprinkle with chopped hazelnuts.

Bircher muesli

2 tbsp whole oats or mixed cereal flakes (barley, spelt, rye, wheat)

1 tbsp lemon juice

3 tbsp water

2 tbsp plain yogurt

1 tsp acacia honey

1 small or ½ large apple, grated

a pinch of cinnamon, finely grated lemon zest (untreated) or freshly grated ginger

1 tbsp chopped nuts (e.g. hazelnuts, almonds, walnuts, pecans, Brazil nuts)

a portion of chopped seasonal fruit (raspberries, strawberries, apricots, peaches, pears, bananas, etc.) or dried fruit (apricots, apples, figs, raisins, goji berries, etc.)

This breakfast dish was pioneered in 1900 by the Swiss doctor Maximilian Bircher-Brenner for patients in his sanatorium, where a diet rich in fresh fruit and vegetables was an essential part of therapy.

In contrast to most conventional shop-bought packaged breakfast cereals, the bulk of this dish comes from fresh fruit, with grains, nuts and yogurt playing tasty supporting roles. Another advantage over dry, boxed cereal lies in the fact that the oats have soaked in water and lemon juice overnight, making them easier to digest. Its wealth of healthy fats, fiber, protein, minerals, vitamins and healthy bacteria makes this a very nourishing start to the day. Serves 1.

Combine oats, lemon juice and water in a container and soak overnight in the refrigerator, tightly covered. If using dried fruits, soak these with the oats to soften them.

Just before eating, add yogurt, honey, grated apple and spices and stir well to combine. If it seems too dry, add some more water or a little milk.

Scatter with freshly cut seasonal fruit and chopped nuts or seeds.

Chocolate Bircher muesli

This isn't exactly Swiss sanatorium fare, but it's a nice variation of the previous recipe and a favorite among chocolate lovers. It's also great in springtime, when apples lose their appeal and fresh summer fruit is slow in showing. Serves 1.

Soak the flakes in water overnight. In the morning, add hazelnut butter, honey, cocoa and yogurt, and stir into a thick paste with a spoon. Add milk (almond or hazelnut) to dilute to desired thickness. Dot with banana slices, scatter with chopped hazelnuts and dust, if you like, with a pinch of cinnamon. Enjoy!

2 tbsp whole oats or mixed cereal flakes

2-3 tbsp water

1 tsp hazelnut butter

½ tsp honey

1 heaped tsp pure cocoa

2 tbsp plain yogurt

splash of nut milk

½ banana, thinly sliced

1 tbsp chopped hazelnuts

Prunella

Inspired by the sugary chocolate-hazelnut paste loved by all children, this healthy remake tastes every bit as chocolatey and hazelnutty but is much lower in sugar as it is sweetened with a mixture of prune puree and honey. Hazelnut butter provides healthy fats and proteins, and the spread is dairy-free. Slather on wholegrain toast, smear onto pancakes, dab on banana slices or stir into yogurt. (This paste is rich in calories, so enjoy sparingly.) Makes about 10oz/1¼ cup/300g.

In a mixing bowl, combine all the ingredients except hazelnut butter and mix. With a metal spoon, carefully fold hazelnut paste into this mixture, taking care not to stir too vigorously or the oil may separate out. Add a little more water if you want a softer paste.

Transfer to an empty, clean jam jar; keeps for about two weeks in the refrigerator.

5¼ oz/⅔ cup/150g hazelnut butter

3.5oz/scant ½ cup/100g prune puree (health-food shop, or Prune sauce p. 261)

2-3 tbsp honey (to taste)

1 heaped tbsp pure, unsweetened cocoa

2-3 tbsp lukewarm water

1 tsp natural vanilla extract

Almond waffles with blueberry sauce

2 eggs

4.5oz/1 ½ cups/125g ground almonds

4.5oz/1 cup/125g whole spelt or wheat flour

1 heaped tsp baking powder

1 tsp natural vanilla extract

10fl oz/1¼ cups/300ml milk (almond, hazelnut, soy or dairy)

pinch of salt

Blueberry sauce

1.1lb/500g blueberries (fresh or defrosted)

pinch of grated lemon zest (untreated)

3.5fl oz/scant ½ cup/100ml berry juice (e.g. blueberry, cherry, raspberry), unsweetened

1 heaped tbsp corn starch

2 tbsp honey

For people trying to wean themselves off processed or starchy breakfast foods, here's a morning dish that's light yet filling and rich in healthy fats and protein to help stabilize blood-sugar levels. These can be made in advance, frozen (separated with baking parchment) and defrosted under the grill. Makes 4-6 waffles, depending on the size of your waffle iron.

Start by making the blueberry sauce (this can be done in advance). Combine juice and corn starch in a medium pot and bring to the boil; stir until the juice has thickened. Remove from heat, add blueberries, lemon zest and honey. Stir well and set aside to cool. Keeps for several days chilled in a tightly sealed container.

In a mixing bowl, combine all the waffle ingredients and whisk until you obtain a smooth, thick batter. Heat waffle iron and bake the waffles as directed by the machine's instructions. Cool for a minute on a wire rack and serve with the blueberry sauce.

Variations
- This recipe works equally well using ground hazelnuts in the place of almonds, hazelnut milk and cinnamon. Topped with apple sauce, this makes a delicious winter breakfast.
- Add 1 teapoon each of pure cocoa powder and honey to the batter for chocolate waffles.

Kousmine-Budwig power breakfast

This recipe is based on the famous "Budwig Cream," a breakfast dish developed by two pioneering European cancer researchers, Catherine Kousmine (1904-1992) and Johanna Budwig (1908-2003). The combination of fruit, cottage cheese or yogurt, nuts, seeds and oil is designed to kick-start the body's detoxification process in the morning. You can either enjoy this chunky, or put all the ingredients in a blender and whizz them into a creamy smoothie. Serves 1.

Whisk cottage cheese or yogurt and oil in a bowl until you obtain a creamy blend. In a small electric blender or chopper, grind the nuts or flaxseed and the cereals. Mash the banana with a fork.

Add all the ingredients, including lemon juice, chopped apple and seasonal fruit, to the yogurt/cheese mix and stir well.

Alternatively, layer ingredients in a tall glass, eat with a long spoon and pretend you're treating yourself to a sundae!

4 tbsp cottage cheese or plain yogurt

2 tbsp walnut oil

1 small banana or 1 tsp raw honey

juice of ½ lemon

pinch of freshly grated ginger or lemon zest (untreated)

2 tbsp freshly ground flax seeds or 6 almonds, walnuts or hazelnuts

2 tbsp whole cereal flakes (e.g. buckwheat, oats)

1 portion seasonal fruit (e.g. apple, pear, strawberries, raspberries, cherries, peach)

Hazelnut-chocolate oatmeal

7oz/scant 1 cup/200ml
hazelnut, almond or soy
milk

2 heaped tbsp small, rolled
oats or other cereal flakes

1 tbsp finely ground
hazelnuts

1 tsp chocolate chips
with 70% cocoa content,
or coarsely chopped
chocolate

½ tsp butter (optional)

Oatmeal porridge can be made with any type of flaked grain such as oats, barley, kamut, spelt, rye or wheat. For optimal digestion and assimilation, the flakes should be soaked in a little water overnight. Soaking speeds up their cooking time in the morning, making this a true "fast food."

This porridge is a very versatile dish that can be adapted to all seasons. Makes 1 serving

Soak flakes overnight in the pot that you plan to use: barely cover with filtered water, cover and leave in a cool place.

When you're ready to prepare the oatmeal, set the pot over medium heat, add milk to the soaked oats and slowly bring to a boil on low heat, stirring to prevent burning. As the mixture thickens, add ground hazelnuts and keep stirring. When the oatmeal has reached the desired thickness, remove from heat. Pour into serving bowl and top with chocolate chips and, if desired, a small pat of butter.

Variations
- Omit chocolate chips and stir half a grated apple, 2 tbsp of apple sauce or stewed fruit into the oatmeal along with a pinch of cinnamon
- In the summer, replace chocoalte chips with 2-3 tbsp mixed berries or fruit *coulis* (p. 261).

Olive oil granola

I know what you're thinking: "Olive oil in my breakfast cereal? Yuck!" Hear me out please. Yes, raw olive oil has quite a strong flavor, but flavored with vanilla, cinnamon, almond butter and a smidgen of honey and baked with whole grains, nuts and dried fruits, all you're left with is but the faintest hint of its herbaceous freshness — and a vat of delicious, crunchy granola!

This quick and easy granola suits people seeking a nutritious, low-sugar alternative to boxed breakfast cereal. Eaten with fresh fruit and/or a dollop of plain yogurt, it should keep you going until lunchtime. Sprinkled on stewed fruit or apple sauce, this crunchy seed-and-grain mix can even double as a crumble topping for a quick, healthy dessert. Makes about 1.1lb/500g of granola.

Preheat oven to 350°F/180°C.

In a large mixing bowl, combine the dry ingredients (except the dried fruit) and mix well.

In a small pot, combine olive oil, honey, nut butter and vanilla extract and warm gently on low heat, stirring with a whisk (do not boil). When it has attained a smooth, glossy texture, remove from heat and pour over dry ingredients.

Mix evenly with an electric whisk and spread out on a large baking tray. Place this in the oven and bake for 30 minutes, stirring every 10-15 minutes to allow even baking.

Remove from oven, add chopped dried fruit and cool; the flakes won't be crunchy when they're warm, but they'll crisp up as they cool. Store in an airtight jar for up to four weeks.

12oz/4⅓ cups/350g whole, organic flakes (e.g. oats, barley, spelt or a mix)

3.5oz/⅔ cup/100g mixed nuts (e.g. almonds, hazelnuts, pecans, cashews, pine nuts), coarsely chopped

3 tbsp mixed seeds (such as pumpkin, sunflower, flax)

1 tsp cinnamon

4 tbsp olive oil

2 tbsp acacia honey

3 tbsp almond or hazelnut butter

2 tsp natural vanilla extract

pinch of salt

3oz/½ cup/75g dried fruit (e.g. raisins, cranberries, cherries, blueberries, chopped apple rings, chopped dried apricots)

Baking

Since most baked goods don't correspond with my definition of "nutrient rich," this section is relatively modest. However, even I love birthday cakes, baked desserts and snacks, and if you put your mind to it, these can be quite nutritious – especially if you avoid using a lot of sugar and replace wheat flour with other ingredients.

One of my favorite flour substitutes are ground almonds or hazelnuts. They produce moist yet light cakes that keep fresh for days and contain substantially more protein, healthy fats and fiber than cakes baked using white flour.

Moreover, they are ideally suited to individuals with gluten allergies: for example, the Queen of Sheba chocolate cake on p. 249 is my standard recipe for children's birthday parties where at least one little guest suffers from a gluten intolerance. This cake tastes so "normal" that no one will even notice the difference!

When you bake, try to make cookies and cakes as nutrient-rich as possible by using nuts, seeds, dried fruits, eggs and spices aplenty and cutting back on excess sugar and fat. These not only taste great; they are also so rich in nutrients that you won't want to eat more than one helping to feel fully satisfied.

Prune flan

A specialty of Brittany on the west coast of France, *Far Breton* is a fruity flan traditionally consisting of a dense, chewy batter with brandy-soaked prunes and raisins nestling beneath. In this healthy version, brandy is replaced with green tea, flour with ground almonds and the batter is delicately perfumed with ginger and lemon zest. The result is a moist, nourishing flan supplying plenty of fiber and protein, and sweetness with a moderate glycemic impact. Makes about thirty 3 by 3 inch/6 by 6 cm squares (gluten-free).

Brew green tea and infuse for 10 minutes.

Preheat oven to 350°F/180°C. Line an approximately 8 by 12 inch/20 by 30 cm ovenproof dish with greaseproof baking paper. Place prunes in a bowl, cover with the hot tea and soak for 30 minutes.

In a mixing bowl, combine ground almonds and corn starch and make a well at the center. Break eggs into this well and stir with a whisk. Gradually add milk and keep stirring until you obtain a smooth, creamy batter. Add ginger, lemon zest, honey and a pinch of salt and mix well.

Add soaked prunes to the batter, stir gently to ensure all fruits are coated and gently pour into the lined baking dish. Scatter with almond slivers and, if desired, with a tablespoonful of raw cane sugar. Bake for 30 minutes or until golden-brown on top and set.

Remove from oven and cool for 15 minutes before cutting into squares.

Variations
- You can use different dried fruit, such as apricots or raisins. Simply replace some or all of the prunes.

---

1 mug (about 11 fl oz/1 cup/330 ml) strong green tea

15oz/400g prunes, halved if very large

7oz/2 1/3 cups/200g finely ground almonds or hazelnuts

2 heaped tbsp corn starch

4 eggs

13½ fl oz/1⅔ cups/400ml almond or other nut milk

1 tsp powdered ginger

finely grated zest of 1 lemon (untreated)

2 tbsp acacia honey

2-3 tbsp almond slivers

pinch of salt

1 tbsp raw cane sugar (optional)

Chocolate-almond *financiers*

3.5oz/100g chocolate (70% cocoa content or more)

3 tbsp olive oil or butter

4 egg whites or 2 whole eggs

3 tbsp acacia honey

4.5oz/1½ cups/125g ground almonds

1 tbsp corn starch

1 tsp natural vanilla extract

1oz/25g dried cherries or cranberries

4 tbsp slivered or chopped almonds

These small French cakes are so delicious, nutritious and filling that one will probably be all you need to satisfy an occasional cake craving. The origin of their name, coined over 100 years ago, is murky; some say it is because only bankers, or financiers, could afford almonds at the time; others claim it's because the traditional rectangular *financier* molds produce cakes in the shape of gold ingots. If you don't have *financier* molds, you can make these in small muffin molds. Makes 10-15 (gluten-free).

Preheat the oven to 350°F/180°C. Lightly grease *financier* or muffin molds.

To melt the chocolate, break it into small pieces and place in a glass or metal bowl with the oil or butter, whichever using. Boil 1 pint/500ml of water and pour carefully into a larger bowl. Set smaller bowl on the hot water and stir until chocolate and fat have blended into a smooth, velvety cream. Remove chocolate and set aside to cool.

In a medium mixing bowl, combine eggs or egg whites (whichever using), honey, ground almonds, corn starch and vanilla and mix well with a fork or a wire whisk. Slowly add melted chocolate and cherries or cranberries and fold in gently.

Spoon the batter into molds. Bake for 10-15 minutes, depending on the size and shape of your molds. The cakes should rise slightly and the surface may crack, but they should feel soft to the touch. Cool for 5 minutes in the molds before turning out on a rack to cool completely. Stored in an airtight container, these keep for about three days.

Sweet potato flan

A great way to wean your taste buds off sugar, this moist and spicy flan is deliciously sweet without containing any added sweetener. It can be enjoyed warm or cold, as a dessert (with Coconut cream, below, if you want to push the boat out), for breakfast or as a sweet snack. Makes one 9-inch/23-cm flan (gluten-free).

Preheat oven to 350°F/180°C. Line the bottom of a round cake tin (9-inch/23-cm diameter) with greaseproof paper and lightly rub the sides with butter.

Steam sweet potatoes for 15-20 minutes; remove from heat.

Meanwhile, warm a dry frying pan on medium heat and toast grated coconut until it turns a light golden color. Tip onto a plate to cool.

Tip soft potatoes into mixing bowl and beat into a soft puree with an electric whisk. Add butter and whisk again to melt. Add eggs, lemon zest, ginger, spices, corn starch, baking powder, dried fruit and salt and whisk thoroughly.

Pour into prepared cake tin and place in preheated oven. Bake for 30-40 minutes, ensuring the top doesn't brown too much; loosely cover with foil if it does. The flan is done when a knife tip inserted in its center comes out clean.

While the flan is baking, prepare Coconut pouring cream (optional). Combine all ingredients in a small bowl and whisk until combined.

Remove flan from oven and leave to cool. Transfer to a cake plate and sprinkle with lightly toasted grated coconut before serving, with or without coconut cream on the side.

1¾ lb/800g sweet potatoes (orange-fleshed), peeled and cubed

2 tbsp lightly toasted grated coconut

2oz/4 tbsp/60g butter

4 eggs

grated zest of ½ lemon (untreated)

½ tsp powdered ginger

1 tsp cinnamon

1 tsp natural vanilla extract

pinch of nutmeg

2 tbsp corn starch

1 tsp baking powder

2oz/ heaped ⅓ cup/60g raisins or dried cranberries

pinch of salt

Coconut pouring cream

7fl oz/scant 1 cup/200ml coconut cream

1 tsp acacia honey

pinch of grated lemon zest (untreated)

1 tsp natural vanilla extract

Chocolate and beet cake

5oz/150g dark chocolate (at least 70% cocoa solids), plus 3 squares (1oz/30 g) of the same chocolate for covering

4 tbsp olive oil or butter

10oz/300g unseasoned beets, cubed (precooked and vacuum-packed)

4 eggs

4 tbsp acacia honey

1 tbsp pure cocoa

1 tsp natural vanilla extract

1 tsp baking powder

1 pinch salt

4.5oz/1½ cups/125g ground almonds

2oz/⅓ cup/60g dried cherries (optional)

2 tbsp grated coconut, roasted almond slivers or chopped hazelnuts to garnish

The French love a dark, gooey chocolate cake, often called *fondant* (melting) or *moelleux* (moist) to reflect its buttery-sugary richness. Here, I use beets for moisture and sweetness, and flour is replaced with ground almonds as the perfect partner for bitter chocolate. Makes one 9-inch/23-cm cake (gluten-free).

Preheat oven to 350°F/180°C. Line the bottom of a 9-inch/23-cm round cake tin with greaseproof paper and grease its sides.

To melt the chocolate, break into small pieces and place in a glass or metal bowl with the oil or butter. Boil 1 pint/500ml of water and pour carefully into a larger bowl. Set smaller bowl on the hot water and stir chocolate as it melts until chocolate and oil/butter have blended into a smooth, velvety liquid. Once fully melted, remove chocolate and set aside.

In a blender, combine beets, eggs, honey, cocoa, vanilla extract, baking powder and salt and whizz until thick and creamy (about 3 minutes). Add almonds and blend to combine. Add chocolate-oil mixture to the batter in the blender and whizz to combine. Add cherries (if using) but do not blend – just stir in with a spoon.

Pour into prepared cake tin and bake in preheated oven for 35-40 minutes. To test for doneness, a skewer inserted into the middle of the cake should come out clean. Remove from oven and place the three squares of chocolate on top of the hot cake; leave to soften and spread over the surface with the back of a teaspoon. Sprinkle with grated coconut, toasted almond slivers or chopped toasted hazelnuts.

This is delicious served with Raspberry *coulis* (p. 261).

Queen of Sheba chocolate cake

If you're not keen on beets in your chocolate cake (previous recipe) you may prefer this luxurious, rich-yet-light French classic, *Gâteau Reine de Saba*. Served with Strawberry or Raspberry coulis (p. 261) or a scoop of Raspberry *semifreddo* (p. 253) it makes the perfect dinner-party dessert; adorned with candles and chocolate sprinkles, it doubles as a delicious gluten-free birthday cake. Makes one 9-inch/23-cm cake (gluten-free).

Preheat oven to 350°F/180°C. Line the bottom of a 9-inch/23-cm cake tin with greaseproof paper and lightly rub the sides with butter.

To melt the chocolate, break it into small pieces and place in a glass or metal bowl with butter, oil and coffee (if using). Boil 1 pint/500ml of water and pour carefully into a larger bowl. Set bowl containing chocolate on the hot water and stir until it has melted into a smooth, velvety liquid. Remove and set aside to cool.

In a large mixing bowl with an electric whisk, beat egg whites until firm. In another bowl, whisk egg yolks and honey until frothy, add chocolate-butter-oil mixture and combine. Add vanilla extract and ground almonds or hazelnuts and whisk into a smooth batter.

Now gently fold in the beaten egg whites, taking care to lift rather than stir them into the batter so that it remains light and airy. Pour batter into cake tin and bake for 30 minutes, or until risen and slightly cracked on top.

Remove cake from oven, cool for 5 minutes in the tin and then turn out onto a cooling rack. Once cooled, transfer to serving plate and dust lightly with dark cocoa powder or icing sugar.

4.5oz/125g dark chocolate (70% cocoa content or more)

3 tbsp soft butter

3 tbsp olive oil

2 tbsp strong espresso coffee (optional)

4 eggs, whites and yolks separated

2-3 tbsp acacia honey

1 tsp natural vanilla extract

3.5oz/1¼ cups/100g ground almonds or hazelnuts

1 tsp pure cocoa powder or icing sugar

Desserts, sweet treats and drinks

If you worry that anti-cancer eating means completely relinquishing desserts and sweet treats, the next section should come as a relief.

Most of us enjoy a bit of sweetness every now and then and it would be unnecessarily draconian to suggest that you banish such tasty treats forever. Industrially manufactured candy and desserts are best avoided, but home-made treats featuring fruits, nuts, chocolate, spices, healthy fats, honey and eggs – such as the ones that follow – are quite another thing.

My general rule regarding dessert is to eat it infrequently – maybe twice a week. Nutritionally speaking, dessert is generally a tasty but not very nutritious optional extra. That's why, on busy weeknights when I barely have enough time to throw together a healthy main meal, it seems pointless to spend time and energy on making dessert. On these occasions a piece of fruit or a square of dark chocolate are enough to satisfy my sweet tooth.

I save "proper" desserts for weekends or guests, when I have more time to prepare and savor them. Given that desserts generally are quite rich in calories, I always make sure that they are also rich in nutrients and that portions sizes are small. Most of us just want "something sweet" after a meal – it doesn't have to be a whole big bowlful!

One very Mediterranean way of ending a meal is simply to nibble on fresh or dried fruits and nuts. I sometimes place a variety of these (e.g., Brazil nuts, almonds and hazelnuts, dried apricots, figs and apples) on a segmented platter of the kind that's often used for salted snacks and let everyone help themselves. Dried fruits stuffed with nuts (see Nuttycots p. 263) are also tasty. Eating out of the same dish as your fellow diners is not only very convivial, it also cuts down on the washing-up!

Very berry summer pudding

It's hard to imagine a more concentrated – or delicious – way of enjoying our red, blue and purple friends, the berries and cherries. This is also a great way to get children to eat berries, which, on their own, they often find too tart. While it is best to eat fruits and vegetables during their local growing season, we can make an exception here: the berry season being woefully short and fresh berries often expensive, I'm happy to make this with frozen berries and enjoy it all year round. Serves 4.

If using frozen berries, scatter onto a large tray or platter and defrost (about 30 minutes).

Pour juice (or juice/wine mixture, whichever using) into a medium pot, add corn starch, lemon zest and honey and mix. Over medium heat, bring the liquid to a simmer, stirring continually with a balloon whisk until it thickens. Remove from heat, tip in the defrosted berries and stir gently with a spoon to coat these evenly with the thickened juice. Adjust sweetness with honey, one spoonful at a time.

Spoon into a glass serving bowl or individual glasses. Decorate with mint leaves and serve at room temperature or chilled.

If you like, you can serve this with Vanilla cashew cream (p. 231) or topped with plain yogurt thinned with a little milk and flavored with honey and vanilla.

1.1lb/500g mixed pitted cherries and berries (raspberries, strawberries, blueberries, cranberries, red- and black currants, blackberries, gooseberries etc.), fresh or frozen

7fl oz/scant 1 cup/200ml cherry or red berry juice (or a combination of 4fl oz/½ cup/120ml juice and 2.5fl oz/⅓ cup/80ml red wine for a more grown-up version)

2 tbsp corn starch

grated zest of ½ lemon (untreated)

3-4 tbsp acacia honey (more or less to taste)

some mint leaves for decoration

Chocolate fondue

fresh seasonal fruit (banana, pineapple, pear, kiwi, tangerine, orange, apricots, strawberries, cherries, bananas, exotic fruits) and/or dried fruit (figs, prunes, apricots)

chopped or grated nuts (almonds, hazelnuts, coconut)

7oz/200g dark chocolate (70% cocoa content or more)

5fl oz/⅔ cup/150ml almond, hazelnut or soy milk

1 tsp natural vanilla extract

juice of ½ lemon

This fun and healthy dessert is quick and easy to prepare and delights diners of all ages. Serves 4.

Cut larger fruits into bite-sized chunks and drizzle with lemon juice to prevent them turning brown. Place on a serving plate, cover and keep cool. Place chopped or grated nuts in a bowl and set aside.

Break chocolate into small pieces. Heat milk in a pot on low heat and when it is about to boil, remove from heat and add chocolate and vanilla extract. Stir energetically with a balloon whisk until the chocolate and milk have melted into a thick, creamy mixture. If it's too thick, add a tablespoon or two of warm milk to dilute.

Pour into a fondue pot and place over a small flame to keep warm. Alternatively, pour chocolate sauce into individual ramekins (pre-warmed), one per person.

To eat, simply skewer the fruit with a fork or bamboo skewer and dip it into the chocolate, and then (if desired) into the chopped nuts for added crunch.

Variations

Once melted, you can flavor the chocolate by adding
- a few spoonfuls of Raspberry *coulis* (p. 261)
- a pinch of cinnamon or cayenne pepper
- a splash of rose water for an exotic touch
- a pinch of orange or lemon zest (untreated) or some drops of their essential oils
- 4-5 tablespoonfuls of strong, freshly brewed tea, such as Earl Grey

Raspberry *semifreddo*

This recipe is inspired by *semifreddo* ("half-cold" in English), a luscious Italian ice cream dessert. Here we replace cream, eggs and sugar with bananas, yogurt and a smidgen of honey. This recipe requires neither an ice-cream maker nor many hours of cooking and chilling time; all you need to do is freeze the banana slices in advance. I usually keep some on stand-by in a small bag in the freezer. Serves 4.

Remove banana slices and berries from the freezer and tip into the food processor. Leave for 10 minutes to soften up. Add honey and yogurt and pulse until creamy.

You may need to stop the processor to scrape frozen bits of fruit off the sides. If the processor gets stuck, wait a few minutes for the ingredients to soften a little and continue processing until the contents have blended into a uniform pink cream.

Enjoy this straight away in its semi-soft state, or freeze and eat later (remove from freezer 10-15 minutes before eating to let it soften).

5oz/150g ripe banana (roughly 2 small bananas) cut into ¼-inch/5-mm slices and frozen on a baking tray lined with parchment paper for at least 1 hour

10oz/300g frozen raspberries (strawberries and blueberries work well, too)

1 tbsp acacia honey (or more to taste)

3.5oz/½ cup/100g plain Greek yogurt

Gingery strawberry relish

zest and juice of ½ orange (untreated)

½ inch/1cm fresh ginger root

½ firm avocado, finely cubed

9oz/1⅔ cups/250g ripe strawberries (untreated)

8 mint leaves

This refreshing and strikingly beautiful blend of fruits tastes great alongside chocolate cake, atop plain yogurt or rice pudding, or simply on its own. Serves 4 as a topping; for full dessert-sized portions, double the quantities.

Place orange zest and juice in a mixing bowl. Peel and finely grate ginger into the bowl. Peel and finely cube avocado and add to bowl. Cut strawberries into quarters and add. Finally, shred 5 mint leaves and add.

Combine everything very gently (be careful not to crush the soft fruit) and leave to infuse in the refrigerator for 1 hour. Serve in individual bowls and sprinkle with remaining chopped mint leaves.

Green tea and ginger egg creams

Fresh and nourishing, this creamy pudding is easy to make and packed with anti-cancer ingredients: ginger, lemon zest, green tea and raspberries. You can use other berries, such as blueberries or strawberries, or enjoy just the custard on its own. Serves 4.

Place raspberries in a small bowl, add 1-2 tablespoons honey (to taste) and mash with a fork. Set aside.

Pour the milk into a small pot, add chopped ginger and lemon zest and bring close to boiling. Remove from heat and infuse for 5 minutes, more if you have time.

Place *matcha* tea in a small cup and add 4 tablespoons hot water. Whisk until smooth and infuse for a few minutes.

Place egg yolks in a small cooking pot. Add corn starch and 2 tablespoons honey and beat with a balloon whisk to combine. Pour infused milk through a fine-meshed sieve onto the egg mixture and whisk to combine. Place on low heat and stir constantly until the cream thickens; remove immediately to avoid the eggs curdling and continue stirring vigorously for 30 seconds. Add infused tea (it will make the custard turn light green).

Cool custard for 10 minutes, then spoon into serving glasses with a large spoon. Top with raspberry puree and chill for at least one hour. Just before serving, sprinkle with chopped mint leaves and/or pistachio nuts.

5¼oz/1 cup/150g raspberries, fresh or frozen (defrosted)

3-4 tbsp acacia honey

13½ fl oz/1⅔ cups/400ml almond, hazelnut or soy milk

1 inch/2cm fresh ginger root, coarsely chopped

finely grated zest of ½ lemon (untreated)

1 tsp matcha *green tea powder* (from specialist tea shops)

4 egg yolks

2 tbsp corn starch

4 mint leaves

2 tbsp chopped pistachio nuts

Chocolate mousse

Mousse

3.5oz/100g dark chocolate (70% cocoa content or more)

15oz/400g silken tofu

1 tbsp acacia honey (more or less, to taste)

½ portion plain Cashew cream (p. 231)

chocolate shavings, cocoa powder or chopped nuts to decorate

Raspberry layers (optional)

5¼oz/1 cup/150g frozen, defrosted raspberries

2 tbsp acacia honey

Most people who taste this for the first time are amazed to learn that it contains none of the usual chocolate mousse ingredients: sugar, eggs, cream or butter. In fact, chocolate, silken tofu and a smidgen of acacia honey are the only ingredients. The texture is just like a traditional mousse, but without the palate-sticking richness. Layered with crushed raspberries and Cashew cream (below), this is elegant enough to serve to dinner guests. Serves 4-5.

To melt the chocolate, break it into small pieces and place in a glass or metal bowl. Boil 1 pint/500ml of water and pour carefully into a larger bowl. Set smaller bowl on the hot water and stir until chocolate has melted into a smooth, velvety liquid. Set aside.

In a blender, whip tofu and honey into a smooth cream. Pour melted chocolate into the tofu cream while blending. Blend the mixture for 3 minutes to incorporate air.

If you want plain chocolate mousse, pour chocolate-tofu cream into ramekins or glasses, cover with plastic food wrap and place in the refrigerator. It becomes fluffier if left to chill for at least 6 hours; eaten earlier, it has a creamy texture.

Just before serving, pour 2-3 tbsp Cashew cream over each mousse and decorate with cocoa powder (cappuccino-style), chocolate shavings or nuts.

Raspberry layers

Layering the mousse with crushed raspberry gives it a fresh, fruity tang. Mash raspberries and honey with a fork and then fill glasses in alternating layers: first raspberry, then chocolate mousse, then more raspberry and chocolate mousse, then top off with a layer of Cashew cream, as above. Adorn with a single raspberry and a light dusting of freshly grated chocolate just before serving.

Cardamom pears in green-tea syrup

A simple, elegant and refreshing dessert to finish a rich meal. Serves 4.

Place pear quarters in a medium pot, add juice, cardamom, ginger, lemon peel and honey, cover and gently bring to the boil. Simmer until pears are soft (5-10 minutes) and remove from heat. Remove pears with a slotted spoon and place in a glass serving bowl.

Separately, whisk 4 tablespoons water with corn starch and green tea until the tea is evenly dispersed and the water has turned green. Combine this with the juice in the pot and bring back to the boil, stirring gently until the juices thicken. Adjust flavoring with lemon juice and honey as necessary.

Pour pale-green syrup over the pears in the bowl and chill for at least 2 hours. Remove ginger slices, lemon peel and cardamom pods before serving.

4 pears, peeled, cored and quartered

12fl oz/1½ cups/350ml pear or apple juice (for an elegant dinner-party dessert, replace 3.5fl oz/100ml of the juice with sweet white wine)

4 cardamom pods

1 inch/2cm fresh ginger root, sliced

2 inch/4cm segment of lemon peel (untreated)

1 tbsp acacia honey

4 tbsp water

1 heaped tsp corn starch

1 tsp matcha green tea

squeeze of lemon juice

Prunes in red wine

1.1lb/500g pitted prunes

8½ fl oz/1 cup/250ml orange juice (freshly pressed if possible)

3.5fl oz/½ cup/100ml red wine

½ tsp ground ginger

grated zest of ½ orange (untreated)

1 cinnamon stick

Happily, the days when people would titter nervously at the mere mention of the word "prune" are over. This modest stone fruit is simply too delicious to be left as an emergency treatment for troubled bowels! This preparation is delicious as dessert (with or without Cashew cream or yogurt) or as a side dish for braised meat or roast duck. It's also great at breakfast, chopped and mixed with muesli or oatmeal, or mashed onto a slice of toast slathered with hazelnut butter. These prunes keep well in a closed container in the refrigerator, so don't hesitate to make more than you think you'll need. Serves 6.

Place prunes in a small pot and cover with orange juice and wine. Add ginger, orange zest and cinnamon stick.

Slowly bring to the boil and simmer for 15 minutes on low heat. Remove from heat and leave prunes to cool in the cooking juices. If the prunes absorb too much juice, add some more water or orange juice (they should sit in a nice, thick syrup).

When fully cooled, transfer to a serving bowl or storage container and chill. Remove from refrigerator 15 minutes before eating.

Green tea and verbena fruit soup

It's hard to imagine a more refreshing and aromatic summer dessert than this. You can make it with any fruit the season offers – strawberries, avocado and melons in early summer, apricots and peaches mid-summer, raspberries, nectarines and blueberries in late summer, or all of the above. Cucumber is the surprise ingredient: it adds crunch and freshness. If you can't get verbena, replace it with mint. Serves 4.

In a small cooking pot, combine green tea leaves, 6 verbena or mint leaves (or teabags) add 10fl oz/1¼ cups/300ml water and heat slowly. Turn off heat when liquid starts to get hot but *before* coming to a boil. Set aside to infuse; after 10 minutes, strain through a fine sieve or cheesecloth, stir in honey and lemon zest and leave to cool.

Meanwhile, chop fruit and cucumber into small cubes. Leave blueberries whole. Chop remaining verbena or mint leaves and add to the fruit. Place all the chopped fruit in a bowl.

Pour green-tea infusion over the chopped fruit and mix very gently so as not to damage the fragile fruit cubes. Chill in refrigerator for at least 1 hour. Just before serving, adjust flavor with lemon juice and honey.

2 tsp green tea leaves

10 leaves fresh verveine (verbena) or mint, or 2 verbena or mint teabags

10fl oz/1 ¼ cups/300ml water

1-2 tbsp acacia honey

finely grated zest of ½ lemon (untreated)

2 ripe but firm peaches

3 ripe but firm apricots

½ cantaloupe melon, deseeded

⅓ cucumber, peeled and deseeded

5oz/1⅔ cups/250g fresh or frozen blueberries

squeeze of lemon juice

Corsican cheesecake

1.1lb/450g ricotta cheese

4 eggs, yolks and whites separated

4 tbsp acacia honey

grated zest of 2 lemons (untreated)

1 tbsp corn starch

1 tsp natural vanilla extract

pinch of salt

This cheesecake by the name of *fiadone* is a specialty of the French Mediterranean island of Corsica, where it is made with fresh ewes' milk curd cheese. Oodles of lemon zest and the absence of pastry make this a delightfully light and tangy dessert or teatime treat. If using very fresh ricotta, this cake can get a bit wet. That's why it's best to surround it with multiple layers of kitchen paper for an hour after baking to drain off excess moisture. Makes one 9-inch/23-cm cake.

Preheat oven to 350°F/180°C. Lightly butter a 9-inch/23-cm round cake tin and line bottom with baking parchment.

Place cheese in a mixing bowl, add egg yolks, honey, lemon zest, corn starch and vanilla extract and whisk into a smooth custard. In another bowl, whisk egg whites until firm, adding salt halfway through, and gently fold into the mixture.

Pour into prepared cake tin and bake at the center of the oven for about 40 minutes, or until the top is golden and a sharp knife inserted into the middle comes out clean.

Remove when cooked and cool for 10 minutes. Now comes a simple juggling trick to drain off excess moisture: lay 6-8 layers of kitchen paper on top of the cake and place a large overturned plate on top. Swiftly flip the whole thing over so the cake now rests atop the kitchen paper, on the plate.

Remove cake tin, peel off greaseproof paper and lay another 6-8 leaves of kitchen paper on the now upward-facing surface of the cake and weigh down with another plate. Leave for 30-60 minutes, allowing excess moisture to drain off into the kitchen paper. When drained, remove top plate and paper, turn upside down again onto final serving platter and peel off the layer of paper that the cake was resting on. Sounds complicated, but it's easy, really!

Serve with Apricot or Raspberry *coulis* (p. 261) or fresh berries.

Fruit *coulis*

Fruit *coulis* (pronounced "coolee") is easy to make, delicious and versatile: stirred into yogurt, poured over ice cream or fruit salad, puddings, waffles and pancakes, whipped into mousses or blended into smoothies, it adds an instant zing of nutrients, flavor and color. I make *coulis* from fresh fruit when it's in season and freeze it in plastic containers or ice-cube trays for small portions. (It makes delicious popsicles too!) In the winter, *coulis* can be made from frozen or dried fruit.

Prune sauce

This is delicious with oatmeal, pancakes, or with savory dishes like roast duck.

7oz/200g dried, pitted prunes

10fl oz/1¼ cup/300ml orange juice or water, or half-half

1 tsp finely grated ginger or 1 tsp cinnamon (optional)

Place prunes and spices (if using) in a small pot and cover with juice or water. Bring to the boil, remove from heat, cover and steep for 1 hour. Liquidize in a blender, adding water if necessary to obtain the desired consistency.

Raspberry coulis

This is easy to make with frozen raspberries and tastes great with chocolate desserts.

1.1lb/500g frozen raspberries, defrosted

2-3 tbsp acacia honey (to taste)

Tip berries into a blender and liquidize. Pour through a fine-meshed sieve to remove the pips. Add honey to taste, one spoon at a time so you don't over-sweeten.

Apricot coulis

Make this during apricot season – it's not nearly as good with frozen or canned apricots.

1.1lb/500g apricots, washed, stoned and quartered

½ vanilla pod, split in half lengthwise

zest of ¼ lemon (untreated)

juice of ¼ lemon

2 tbsp acacia honey

Place apricots in a pot and add the remaining ingredients. Bring slowly to the boil and stew on low heat until the apricots are soft. Remove vanilla pod and scrape the black seeds into the stewed fruit. Now tip into blender and liquidize. If the apricots are stringy, pass through a sieve; if not, use straight away.

"Pruffles"

3.5oz/100g dark chocolate (70% cocoa content or more)

2oz/50g hazelnut or almond butter

5¼ oz/150g prunes (pitted)

2 tbsp acacia honey

1 tsp natural vanilla extract

Optional added flavorings

essential oil of orange (2-3 drops)

a pinch of grated fresh ginger or finely chopped candied ginger

cinnamon (1 level tsp)

Coating

pure cocoa powder

finely chopped hazelnuts or walnuts

grated coconut, lightly toasted

Prunes and chocolate have a close affinity. Indeed, in the sleepy town of Agen – the epicenter of France's prune production – every souvenir shop sells prune-and-chocolate confectionery such as these truffles, and local restaurants serve delectable prune-and-chocolate desserts. You can add ginger, orange or cinnamon as flavor enhancers. Makes about 20-25 pruffles.

To melt the chocolate, break it into small pieces and place in a glass or metal bowl along with the nut butter. Boil 1 pint/500ml water and pour carefully into a larger bowl. Set smaller bowl on the hot water and stir gently until chocolate and nut butter have melted into a smooth, velvety cream. Set aside.

Place prunes in a small food processor and blend into a smooth paste. Add honey and vanilla extract and pulse again until smooth. If the mixture is too sticky, add 1-2 tbsp water to soften it up.

Add prune mixture to the melted chocolate and mix thoroughly. Add any additional flavorings (e.g. cinnamon, orange oil or ginger) now. Transfer to a sealable container and chill for at least 2 hours.

Once the mixture has set, scoop out small portions with a teaspoon or melon scoop and shape them into small balls. Toss in cocoa or roll in chopped nuts to coat. Place in refrigerator for at least one hour before serving. These should keep in the refrigerator for up to a week.

Nuttycots

My children invented this during a long car journey. The only snacks available at the time being dried apricots and a packet of walnut halves, they played a rousing game of "guess where I hid the nut" – and thus Nuttycots were born!

Serve these pretty parcels with after-dinner tea and enjoy the contrast of chewy fruit and crunchy nut. Walnuts are my favorites, but pecans, cashews, Brazils or hazelnuts work equally well.

This also makes a convenient lunchbox filler or snack at work. Nuttycots can be made in large batches (a fun rainy Sunday-afternoon activity for children – easy and not too messy) and stored in a tightly sealed container for up to three weeks. Dipped in melted dark chocolate (rather messier!), they make a decadent treat.

If possible, use sulfite-free apricots (sulfites can cause allergic reactions), which are available at health-food shops. Compared to their bright-orange sulfured cousins they have a mellower toffee flavor. If you're bothered by their brownish hue, rub their skins lightly with a drop of olive oil, which gives them a gentle amber glow.

In pitted apricots, a small slit has already been cut to remove the stone. Find this opening, tear slightly to unfold and flatten the apricot, insert nut(s) and fold the flap shut again, partially or completely.

Done!

Make as many as you like, using:

dried, pitted apricots (unsulfured)

mixed nuts (e.g. walnut, pecan, hazelnut, Brazil, cashew)

Cocoa concoctions

As we saw in Chapter 4, unsweetened cocoa powder – as tasty as chocolate but lower in calories – is a great way to obtain health-promoting polyphenols. Here, I suggest two satisfying dairy-free cocoa drinks – one cold, one hot.

Cocoa cooler

We generally associate cocoa with steaming cupfuls of milky comfort on cold winter days, but chilled cocoa can be surprisingly thirst-quenching in warm weather. Here's a refreshing and invigorating drink my husband sometimes makes on hot summer afternoons. For 1 large cup (about 5fl oz/⅔ cup/150ml).

2 tsp high-quality unsweetened cocoa powder

1 tsp honey

2-3 tbsp hot water

4¼fl oz/½ cup/125ml ice-cold water

1 ice cube (optional)

3 drops of essential oil of mint (optional)

In a cup, combine cocoa powder, hot water and honey and stir into a paste. Top up with cold water, add essential oil of mint (if using), whisk with a small spoon or fork and add an ice cube to chill. Serve immediately, decorated perhaps with a mint leaf.

Aztec elixir

This spicy drink will warm you right through to the tips of your toes. If you like it thick, add ½ teaspoon corn starch to the cocoa mix to yield a velvety and comforting beverage you can savor by the spoonful. For 1 large cup (about 5fl oz/⅔ cup/150ml).

2 tsp high-quality unsweetened cocoa powder

½ tsp corn starch (if using)

generous pinch of cinnamon

5 drops natural vanilla extract

pinch of cayenne pepper (optional)

pinch of orange zest (untreated only)

4¼fl oz/½ cup/125ml boiling water

1 tsp honey

In a large mug, mix cocoa powder, corn starch (if using) and spices. Add boiling water and stir with a small whisk or fork until the mixture thickens. Serve immediately.

Green and white tea

If you find plain green or white tea hard to swallow (they can be quite bitter), here are some ideas for turning them into refreshing, easy-drinking beverages you can sip throughout the day. Each recipe yields a 10fl oz/1 ¼ cup/300ml mug.

Green zinger
Enjoy warm or cold. In the summer, triple quantity and chill for delicious iced tea.

---
1 heaped tsp or 1 tea bag green tea

10fl oz/1 ¼ cup/300ml just boiled water

---
thin strip of untreated lemon peel (about 2 inches/4 cm)

---
juice of ½ lemon

---
1 tsp honey

Place tea (in cotton mesh tea infuser) and lemon peel in a large mug. Pour hot water over these and infuse for 8-10 minutes. Remove tea, add lemon juice and honey.

Minty magic
Along the Mediterranean shores of North Africa, strong minty green tea is drunk throughout the day. It is especially a drink of hospitality, served whenever there are guests. Traditionally, the tea is boiled and intensely sweet; here, we go for a lighter, fresher version.

---
1 heaped tsp or 1 tea bag green or white tea

---
1 heaped tbsp chopped fresh mint leaves or 1 mint teabag

10fl oz/1 ¼ cup/300ml water, just boiled

---
1 tsp honey

Place tea and mint leaves or tea bag in a cotton tea infuser and place in a large mug. Cover with hot water and infuse for 10 minutes. Remove tea, add honey and serve.

Green-tea chai
Indian chai is a delicious way of enjoying spices and tea. The spice mix below is my favorite but you can add other spices such as saffron, pepper, coriander, allspice, vanilla, fennel, mace, nutmeg, star anise and even fresh lemongrass.

5fl oz/⅔ cup/150ml water

5fl oz/⅔ cup/150ml almond milk

---
1 crushed cardamom pod, 1 clove, a large pinch each of ground cinnamon, powdered ginger, grated nutmeg

---
1 heaped tsp green/white tea, or 1 tea bag

---
pinch finely grated lemon zest (untreated)

---
1 tsp honey

In a small pot combine water, almond milk and spices and bring to the boil; simmer for 5 minutes on low heat. Remove from heat and add green tea and lemon zest, stir and infuse another 5 minutes. Strain, add honey and enjoy hot or chilled.

Appendix 1 Measurement conversions

Solid measurements

Metric (European)	Imperial (UK and US)
1 kilogram (kg)	2.2 pound (lb)
500 grams (g)	1.1lb
450 g	1lb
200 g	7 ounces (oz)
100 g	3½ oz
60 g	2 oz/4 tablespoons (tbsp)

Liquid measurements

Metric	American
1 liter	2.1 pints / 34 fluid ounces (fl oz)/4¼ cups
500 milliliter (ml)	1 pint or 2 cups
250 ml	½ pint / 8½ fluid ounces / 1 cup
120 ml	4 fl oz / ½ cup
100 ml	3½ fl oz / scant ½ cup
75 ml	2½ fl oz / ⅓ cup
60 ml	2 fl oz / ¼ cup

Oven temperatures

° Celsius	° Fahrenheit	Gas Mark	Description
90	190	¼	Cool
120	250	½	Very slow
140	280	1	Slow
150	300	2	Slow
160	320	3-4	Moderately slow
180	350	4-5	Moderate
190	375	5-6	Moderately hot
200	400	6-8	Hot

Appendix 2 Glossary of culinary terms

I have used American spellings and terminology throughout the book; this international glossary will hopefully help to avoid any misunderstandings.

US terms	British/Australian terms
baked potato	jacket potato
baking soda	bicarbonate of soda
beet	beetroot
blueberry	bilberry
bouillon cube	stock cube
canola oil	rapeseed oil
celery rib	celery stick
cheesecloth	muslin
cilantro	coriander (fresh)
cookies	biscuits
cornstarch	cornflour
dessert	pudding
eggplant	aubergine
extract (e.g. vanilla)	essence
fava beans	broad beans
French fries	chips
granola	muesli
ground meat	minced meat
green beans	French beans
green/spring onion	salad onion
navy beans	haricot beans
peanut	ground nut
popsicle	ice lolly
pot	saucepan
potato chips	crisps
raisins	sultanas
seeds	pips
skillet	frying pan
strainer	sieve
tomato paste	tomato puree
vanilla bean	vanilla pod
zucchini	courgette

Appendix 3 Weeky meal planner

	Monday	Tuesday	Wednesday	Thursday	Friday	Saturday	Sunday
Breakfast							
Snack							
Lunch							
Snack							
Dinner							

Appendix 4 Shopping list

Tick or underline the foods you need, specifying quantity. Write any additional items in the blank spaces.

Fruits and vegetables

(Buy local and seasonal produce; don't buy too much at once as storage reduces nutritional value.

Fresh foods (refrigerator)

- ☐ Omega-3-rich eggs
- ☐ Meat / fish
- ☐ Plain yoghurt
- ☐ Milk / butter / cheese from grass-fed animals (in moderation)
- ☐ Nuts and seeds (walnuts, cashews, Brazils, hazelnuts, almonds, pumpkin seeds, etc.)
- ☐ Tofu requiring refrigeration (e.g. silken tofu, plain firm tofu)
- ☐ Cold pressed oil (e.g. walnut)
- ☐ Sauces / spreads
- ☐
- ☐
- ☐

Frozen foods

- ☐ Frozen berries (e.g. blueberries, raspberries, berry mixes)
- ☐ Other frozen fruit (e.g. apricots, peaches, mangoes, etc.)
- ☐ Frozen vegetables (e.g. peas, beans, carrots, broccoli, cauliflower, leaf spinach, onions, artichoke hearts, plain grilled peppers and eggplant slices, etc.)

Store cupboard items, dry goods

- ☐ Dried beans and lentils
- ☐ Herbs (specify)
- ☐ Spices (specify)
- ☐ Salt, pepper
- ☐ Dried fruit (prunes, apricots, apple rings, cherries, blueberries, etc.)
- ☐ Tea, coffee
- ☐ Dried mushrooms
- ☐ 100% cocoa powder
- ☐ Dark chocolate (70% cocoa content or more)
- ☐ Whole grains (e.g. barley, spelt, oats, etc.)
- ☐ Whole flakes
- ☐ Flour (e.g. spelt, wheat, corn, etc.)
- ☐ Wholegrain pasta
- ☐
- ☐
- ☐

Store cupboard items (in jars, cartons, tins or bottles)

- ☐ Milk & cream (nut/soy/dairy)
- ☐ Soy sauce, balsamic or red wine vinegar
- ☐ Unsweetened coconut milk and cream
- ☐ Beans, tomatoes, mushrooms, olives etc) in jars
- ☐ Pesto, salsa, tapenade (minimally processed)
- ☐ Sundried tomatoes,
- ☐ Tomato concentrate
- ☐ Unsweetened fruit compotes
- ☐ Fruit spreads without added sugar
- ☐ Fish (sardines, mackerel, herring, anchovy) in cans or jars
- ☐
- ☐
- ☐

Appendix 5 Resources

Information on cancer and its prevention

American Institute for Cancer Research
(Part of the WCRF Global Network)
1759 R Street NW
Washington, DC 20009
United States
Tel: +1-202-328-7744
Fax: +1-202-328-7226
Website: www.aicr.org

World Cancer Research Fund (UK)
Second Floor, 22 Bedford Square
London WC1B 3HH
United Kingdom
Tel: +44-20-7343 4200
Fax: +44-20-7343 4220
Website : www.wcrf-uk.org

National Cancer Institute (NCI) of the **U.S. National Institutes of Health**
NCI Office of Communications and Education
Public Inquiries Office
6116 Executive Boulevard
Suite 300
Bethesda, MD 20892-8322
Tel: +1-800-422-6237
Website: www.cancer.gov

Cancer Research UK
P.O. Box 123
Lincoln's Inn Fields
London WC2A 3PX
Tel: (Support Services) 020 7121 6699
Tel: (Switchboard) 020 7242 0200
Fax: 020 7121 6700
Website: www.cancerresearchuk.org
Patient information website:
www. cancerhelp.org.uk

Dietary cancer prevention reading

WCRF/AICR Expert Report can be ordered via the organizations' websites (above).
Anticancer – A New Way of Life, David Servan-Schreiber (Viking 2009)
Foods to Fight Cancer, Richard Béliveau and Denis Gingras (Dorling Kindersley, 2007)
Life Over Cancer, Keith Block M.D. (Bantam 2009)
The Genesis Breast Cancer Prevention Diet, Dr Michelle Harvey (Rodale, 2006)

Mediterranean diet information

Oldways Trust
266 Beacon Street
Boston, MA 02116
Tel: +1-617-421-5500
Fax: +1-617-421-5511
Website: www.oldwayspt.org

Mediterranean diet cook books

There are so many it's impossible to list them all. Here are a few of my favorites:

The French Don't Diet Plan: 10 Simple Steps to Stay Thin for Life by Dr. Will Clower (Three Rivers Press, US; 2006).
Elizabeth David Classics: Mediterranean Food, French Country Cooking and Summer Cooking by Elizabeth David (Grub Street; 1999).
Conquer Diabetes and Prediabetes: The Low-Carb Mediterranean Diet by Dr. Steve Parker, MD (pxHealth, US; 2011)
The New Mediterranean Diet Cookbook by Nancy Harmon Jenkins (Bantam 2009)
Little Foods of the Mediterranean: 500 Fabulous Recipes for Antipasti, Tapas, Hors d'Oeuvres, Meze and More by Clifford A. Wright (Harvard Common Press, US; 2003)

Notes and references

Introduction

1   Based on data in the World Cancer Report 2008 published by the W.H.O.'s International Agency for Research on Cancer, and on a personal communication from Professor Bernard Stewart, University of New South Wales.

2   For more information on the complete range of lifestyle measures that help to reduce cancer risks, visit the websites of the World Cancer Research Fund UK (http://www.wcrf-uk.org/) and the American Institute for Cancer Research (http://www.aicr.org); both are part of the World Cancer Research Fund International (http://www.wcrf.org/).

3   For a discussion of selected scientific studies on the benefits of the Mediterreanean diet, visit the website of the Oldways Trust, a non-profit organization promoting the traditional Mediterranean diet. http:// www.oldwayspt.org/scientific-studies-mediterraneandiet

4   From http://www.wcrf-uk.org/preventing_cancer/recommendations.php

Chapter 1

1   World Cancer Research Fund and American Institute for Cancer Research, *Food, Nutrition, Physical Activity and the Prevention of Cancer: a Global Perspective.* Washington DC, 2007.

2   Donaldson MS, *Nutrition and cancer: A review of the evidence for an anti-cancer diet.* Nutrition Journal 2004, 3:19.

3   Ornish D, Weidner G, Fair WR et al, *Intensive lifestyle changes may affect the progression of prostate cancer.* Journal of Urology, 174(3), 2005: 1065-9; discussion 9-70.

4   Hayat MJ, Howlader N, Reichman ME, Edwards BK, *Cancer Statistics, Trends, and Multiple Primary Cancer Analyses from the Surveillance, Epidemiology, and End Results (SEER) Program.* The Oncologist, Vol. 12, No. 1, 2037, January 2007

5   Adams J, White M, *Socio-economic and gender differences in nutritional content of foods advertised in popular UK weekly magazines.* Eur J Public Health, 2009. Jan 18.

Chapter 2

1   Kouris-Blazos A, Gnardellis C, Wahlqvist ML, Trichopoulos D, Lukito W, Trichopoulou A, *Are the advantages of the Mediterranean diet transferable to other populations? A cohort study in Melbourne, Australia.* British Journal of Nutrition 1999;82:57-61.

2   Lagiou P, Trichopoulos D, Sandin S, Lagiou A, Mucci L, Wolk A, Weiderpass E, Adami H-O, *Mediterranean dietary pattern and mortality among young women: a cohort study in Sweden.* British Journal of Nutrition 2006;96:384-392.

3   Mitrou PN, Kipnis V, Thiébaut ACM, Reedy J, Subar A et al. *Mediterranean dietary pattern and prediction of all-cause mortality in a US population. Arch Intern Med 2007; Vol 167(22): 2461-2468.*

4   Trichopoulou A, Lagiou P, Kuper H, Trichopoulos D, *Cancer and Mediterranean Dietary Traditions.* Cancer Epidemiology, Biomarkers & Prevention. 2000; 9: 869–873.

5   Benetou V, Trichopoulou A, Orfanos P, Naska A, Lagiou P, Boffetta P, Trichopoulos D, *Conformity to traditional Mediterranean diet and cancer incidence: the Greek EPIC cohort.* British Journal of Cancer 2008.*99:191-195.*

6   Knoops, K.T.B., et al, *Mediterranean Diet, Lifestyle Factors, and 10-Year Mortality in Elderly European Men and Women - The HALE Project.* JAMA, 2004. 292: p. 1433-1439.

7   De Lorgeril M, Salen P, Martin J-L, Monjaud I, Boucher P, Mamelle N, *Mediterranean dietary pattern in a randomised trial ; prolonged survival and possible reduced cancer rate.* Arch Int Med 1998;158(11)

8   Benetou V, Orfanos P, Lagiou P, Trichopoulos D, Boffetta P, Trichopoulou A, *Vegetables and fruits in relation to cancer risk: evidence from the Greek EPIC cohort study.* Cancer Epidemiol Biomarkers Prev 2008;17(2).

9   United States Department of Agriculture Economic Research Service, http://www.ers.usda.gov/Data/Food Consumption/2007 data, after adjusting for plate waste, spoilage, and other losses.

10   World Cancer Research Fund/American Institute for Cancer Research, *Food, Nutrition, Physical Activity and the Prevention of Cancer: a Global Perspective.* Washington DC, 2007.

11   Sinha R, et al, *Meat Intake and Mortality.* Archives of Internal Medicine, 2009. 169: p. 562-571.

12   Fernandez E, Chatenoud L, La Vecchia C, Negri E, Franceschi S, *Fish consumption and cancer risk.* Am J Clin Nutr. 1999 Jul;70(1):85-90.

13   Norat T et al, *Meat, fish and colorectal cancer risk: the European prospective investigation into cancer and nutrition.* Journal of the National Cancer Institute 2005. Vol 97(12):906-916.

14   Lucenteforte E, Garavello W, Bosetti C, Talamini R, Zambon P, Franceschi S, et al. *Diet diversity and the risk of squamous cell esophageal cancer.* Int J Cancer 2008;123:2397-2400.

15   Fernandez E, D'Avanzo B, Negri E, Franceschi S, La Vecchia C. *Diet diversity and the risk of colorectal cancer in northern Italy.* Cancer Epidemiol Biomarkers Prev 1996 Jun;5(6):433-6.

16   Garaveto W, Giordano L, Bosetti C, Talamini R, Negri E, Tavain A, et al. *Diet diversity and the risk of oral and pharyngeal cancer.* Eur J Nutr 2008;47:280-284.

17   Ghadirian P, Narod S, Fafard E, Costa M, Robidoux A, Nkondjock A. *Breast cancer risk in relation to the joint effect of BRCA mutations and diet diversity.* Breast Cancer Res Treat 2009 Jan 23.

18   Pollan M. *In Defence of Food,* Penguin Books 2008. The study, commissioned by industry and unpublished, was conducted by John Nihoff, a professor of gastronomy at the Culinary Institute of America.

19   http://www.hagerty.com/NewsManager/templates/template_press.aspx?articleid=420&zoneid=57

20   "From Table Snobs to Caveman Slobs", 12 Oct. 2006. A survey commissioned by 'Great British Chicken', a marketing body associated with the British National Farmers' Union.

21   Pollan M. *In Defence of Food,* Penguin Books 2008. 22 Fischler C, Masson E. *Manger – Français, Européens et Américains face à l'alimentation.* Odile Jacob (Paris), 2008.

Chapter 3

1   IARC press release 1 June 2010, www.iarc.fr/en/ media-centre/pr/2010/pdfs/pr201_E.pdf

2   Hayat MJ, Howlader N, Reichman ME, Edwards BK. *Cancer Statistics, Trends, and Multiple Primary Cancer Analyses from the Surveillance, Epidemiology, and End Results (SEER) Program.* The Oncologist, Vol. 12, No. 1, 2037, January 2007.

3   Kaatsch P, Steliarova-Foucher E, Crocetti E et al, *Time trends of cancer incidence in European children (1978-1997): report from the Automated Childhood Cancer Information System project.* Eur J Cancer. 2006 Sep;42(13):1961-71.

4   Stiller CA, Desandes E, Danon SE et al, *Cancer incidence and survival in European adolescents (1978-1997). Report from the Automated Childhood Cancer Information System project.* Eur J Cancer. 2006 Sep;42(13):2006-18.

5   Cordain L, Eaton SB, Sebastian A et al. *Origins and evolution of the western diet: health implications for the 21st century.* American Journal of Clinical Nutrition 81(2), 2005:341-54.

6   Cordain L, Eaton SB, Sebastian A et al. *Origins and evolution of the western diet: health implications for the 21st century.* American Journal of Clinical Nutrition 81(2), 2005:341-54.

7   World per capita consumption of sugar, 2002 to 2008; International Sugar Organization, London.

8   WCRF/AICR: Food, Nutrition, Physical Activity and the Prevention of Cancer, Washington 2007.

9   Grothey A, Voigt W, Schober C, Muller T, Dempke W, Schmoll HJ, *The role of insulin-like growth factor I and its receptor in cell growth, transformation, apoptosis, and chemoresistance in solid tumours.* J Cancer Res Clin Oncol 1999; 125(3-4):166-73.

10 Sieri S, Pala V, Brighenti F, et al, *Dietary glycemic index, glycemic load, and the risk of breast cancer in an Italian prospective cohort study.* Am J Clin Nutr. 2007;86(4):11601166.

11 Silvera SA, Jain M, Howe GR, Miller AB, Rohan TE, *Dietary carbohydrates and breast cancer risk: a prospective study of the roles of overall glycemic index and glycemic load.* Int J Cancer. 2005;114(4):653-658.

12 Higginbotham S, Zhang ZF, Lee IM, Cook NR, Buring JE, Liu S, *Dietary glycemic load and breast cancer risk in the Women's Health Study.* Cancer Epidemiol Biomarkers Prev. 2004;13(1):65-70.

13 Michaud DS, Fuchs CS, Liu S, Willett WC, Colditz GA, Giovannucci E, *Dietary glycemic load, carbohydrate, sugar and colorectal cancer risk in men and women.* Cancer Epidemiology, Biomarkers & Prevention 2005;14(1):138-47.

14 Augustin LSA, Polesel J, Bosetti C et al, *Dietary glycemic index, glycemic load and ovarian cancer risk: a case-control study in Italy.* Annals of Oncology 2003;14(1):78-84.

14a Stocks T, Rapp K, Bjørge T et al; *Blood glucose and risk of incident and fatal cancer in the metabolic syndrome and cancer project (me-can): analysis of six prospective cohorts.* PLoS Med. 2009 Dec;6(12).

15 Jonas CR, McCullough ML, Teras LR, Walker-Thurmond KA, Thun MJ, Calle EE, *Dietary glycemic index, glycemic load, and risk of incident breast cancer in postmenopausal women.* Cancer Epidemiol Biomarkers Prev. 2003;12(6):573-577.

16 Nielsen TG, Olsen A, Christensen J, Overvad K, Tjonneland A, *Dietary carbohydrate intake is not associated with the breast cancer incidence rate ratio in postmenopausal Danish women.* J Nutr. 2005;135(1):124-128.

17 Giles GG, Simpson JA, English DR, et al, *Dietary carbohydrate, fibre, glycemic index, glycemic load and the risk of postmenopausal breast cancer.* Int J Cancer. 2006;118(7):1843-1847.

18 Lajous M, Boutron-Ruault MC, Fabre A, Clavel-Chapelon F, Romieu I, *Carbohydrate intake, glycemic index, glycemic load, and risk of postmenopausal breast cancer in a prospective study of French women.* Am J Clin Nutr. 2008;87(5):1384-1391.

19 For more detail, the University of Sydney in Australia keeps the most complete database of foods and their GI/GL factors at www.glycemicindex.com.)

20 Pollan M: In Defence of Food, Penguin Books 2008; p. 167

21 Simopoulos AP, *The importance of the ratio of omega-6/omega-3 essential fatty acids.* Biomed Pharmacother. 2002 Oct;56(8):365-79.

22 Innis S, *Dietary Omega 3 and Omega 6 Fatty Acids,* Eds. Gallic , Simopoulos AP, NATO ASI Series, 171 : 142, 1989.

23 Simopoulos, AP and Norman Salem, *Omega-3 fatty acids in eggs from range-fed Greek chickens.* New England Journal of Medicine 1989; 321(20):1412.

24 Slots T, Butler G, Leifert C, *Potentials to differentiate milk composition by different feeding strategies.* J Dairy Sci. 2009 May;92(5):2057-66.

25 Kelley NS, Hubbard NE, Erickson KL, *Conjugated Linoleic acid isomers and cancer.* Journal of Nutrition 2007;137(12):2599-607.

26 Sikorski AM, Hebert N, Swain RA, *Conjugated Linoleic Acid (CLA) inhibits new vessel growth in the mammalian brain.* Brain Res. 2008 Jun 5;1213:35-40. Epub 2008 Feb 16.

27 Butler G, Nielsen JH, Slots T, Seal C,Eyre MD, Sanderson R, Leifert C, *Fatty acid and fat-soluble antioxidant concentrations in milk from high- and low-input conventional and organic systems: seasonal variation.* J Sci Food Agric 2008; 88:1431–1441.

28 Commission of the European Communities, White Paper Strategy for a future Chemicals Policy, 2001. http://eur-lex.europa.eu/LexUriServ/LexUriServ. do?uri=COM:2001:00 88:FIN:en:PDF

29 United States Environmental Protection Agency, Pesticides Industry Sales and Usage: 2000 and 2001 Market Estimates. http://www.epa.gov/oppbead1/pestsales/01pestsales/market_estimates2001.pdf

30 USDA Pesticide Data Program, Annual Summary, Calendar Year 2007 (published December 2008). www. ams.usda.gov/pdp

31 Curl CL, Fenske RA, Elgethun K, *Organophosphorus pesticide exposure of urban and suburban pre-school children with organic and conventional diets.* Environmental Health Perspectives 2003;111(3):377-82.

32 Data retrieved on 3 March 2011 from the Environmental Working Group's website: www.foodnews.org/fulllist.php

33 WCRF/AICD. *Food, Nutrition, Physical Activity and the Prevention of Cancer: a Global Perspective.* Washington DC, 2007.

34 Smith JS, Ameri F, Gadgil P, *Effect of marinades on the formation of heterocyclic amines in grilled beef steaks.* J Food Sci 2008 Aug;73(6):T100-5

35 WCRF/AICR. *Food, Nutrition, Physical Activity and the Prevention of Cancer: A Global Perspective.* Washington DC, 2007.

36 LaPensee EW, Tuttle TR, Fox SR, Ben-Jonathan N, *Bisphenol A at Low Nanomolar Doses Confers Chemoresistance in Estrogen Receptor Alpha Positive and Negative Breast Cancer Cells.* Environ Health Perspect 2008:doi: 10.1289/ehp.11788 (available at http:// dx.i.org/).

37 Yang CZ, Yaniger SI, Jordan VC, Klein DJ, Bittner GD. *Most Plastic Products Release Estrogenic Chemicals: A Potential Health Problem That Can Be Solved.* Environmental Health Perspectives Jul 2011;119(7):989-996.

Chapter 4

1 Dietary chemoprevention is explained in great detail and clarity in *Foods to Fight Cancer.* Béliveau R, Gingras D (Dorling Kindersley, 2007)

2 Chu M, Seltzer TF, *Myxedema coma induced by ingestion of raw bok choy.* N Engl J Med. 2010 May 20;362(20):1945-6.

3 Doerge DR, Sheehan DM, *Goitrogenic and estrogenic activity of soy isoflavones.* Environ Health Perspect. 2002 Jun;110 Suppl 3:349-53.

4 Craig WJ, *Health effects of vegan diets.* Am J Clin Nutr. 2009 May;89(5):1627S-1633S.

5 Burgos-Moron E, Calderon-Montano JM et al, *The dark side of curcumin.* Int J Cancer 2009;126:1771-1775.

6 Lopez-Lazaro M, *Anticancer and carcinogenic properties of curcumin: considerations for its clinical development as a cancer chemopreventive and chemotherapeutic agent.* Mol Nutr Food Res 2008;52(Suppl 1):S103-27.

7 Somasundaram S, Edmund NA, Moore DT et al, *Dietary curcumin inhibits chemotherapy-induced apoptosis in models of human breast cancer.* Cancer Res 2002;67:3853-75.

8 Cao J, JIa L, Zhou HM et al, *Mitochondrial and nuclear DNA damage induced by curcumin in human hepatoma G2 cells.* Toxicol Sci 2006;91:476-83.

9 Jiao Y, Wilkinson J, Di X, et al, *Curcumin, a cancer chemopreventive and chemotherapeutic agent, is a biologically active iron chelator.* Blood 2009. 113 (2): 462–9.

10 Bowman SA, Spence JT, *A Comparison of Low-Carbohydrate vs. High-Carbohydrate Diets: Energy Restriction, Nutrient Quality and Correlation to Body Mass Index.* J Am Coll Nutr 2002; 21(3):268-274.

11 WCRF/AICR, *Policy and Action for Cancer Prevention.* Washington DC, 2009.

12 Fahey JW et al, *Broccoli sprouts: an exceptionally rich source of inducers of enzymes that protect against chemical carcinogens.* Proceedings of the National Academy of Sciences 1997;94;10367-72.

13 Boffetta P et al, *Fruit and vegetable intake and overall cancer risk in the European Prospective Investigation into Cancer and Nutrition (EPIC).* J Natl Cancer Inst. 2010 Apr 21;102(8):529-37.

14 Table translated from Béliveau R, Gingras D, *La santé pour le plaisir de bien manger.* Editions Trécarré 2008.

15 Michels Blanck H, Gillespie C, Kimmons JE, Seymour JD, Serdula MK, *Trends in fruit and vegetable consumption among U.S. men and women, 1994-2005.* Prev Chronic Dis 2008;5(2): A35.

16 *Health of Britain – Perspective on Nutrition 2008*, TNS World Panel, September 2008. http://www.tnsglobal.com/_assets/files/TNS_Market_Research_shape__ of_Britain(1).pdf

17 Tamers SL, Agurs-Collins T, Dodd KW, Nebeling L, *US and France adult fruit and vegetable consumption patterns: an international comparison.* European Journal of Clinical Nutrition 2009;63: 11-17.

18 Galeone C, Pelucchi C, Levi F, La Vecchia C, *Onion and garlic use and human cancer.* American Journal of Clinical Nutrition, Vol. 84, No. 5, 1027-1032.

19 Iciek M, Kwiecie I, Włodek L. *Biological properties of garlic and garlic-derived organosulfur compounds.* Environ Mol Mutagen. 2009 Apr;50(3):247-65.

20 Anna A. Powolny and Shivendra V. Singh, *Multitargeted prevention and therapy of cancer by diallyl trisulfide and related Allium vegetable-derived organosulfur compounds.* Cancer Lett. 2008 October 8; 269(2): 305–314.

21 Milton, K, *Nutritional characteristics of wild primate foods: Do the natural diets of our closest living relatives have lessons for us?* Nutrition 1999, 15(6): 488-498.

22 Monro J, *Treatment of cancer with mushroom products.* Arch Environ Health. 2003 Aug;58(8):533-7.

23 Yang P, Liang M, Zhang Y, Shen B, *Clinical application of a combination therapy of lentinan, multi-electrode RFA and TACE in HCC.* Adv Ther 2008; 25 (8): 787–94.

24 Nakano H, Namatame K, Nemoto H, *A multi-institutional prospective study of lentinan in advanced gastric cancer patients with unresectable and recurrent diseases: effect on prolongation of survival and improvement of quality of life.* Hepatogastroenterology 1999; 46 (28): 2662–8.

25 Hazama S, Watanabe S, Ohashi M, *et al. Efficacy of Orally Administered Superfine Dispersed Lentinan ({beta}1,3-Glucan) for the Treatment of Advanced Colorectal Cancer. Anticancer Res 2009;* 29 (7): 2611–7.

26 Zhang M, Huang J, Xie X, Holman CD, *Dietary intakes of mushrooms and green tea combine to reduce the risk of breast cancer in Chinese women.* Int J Cancer. 2009 Mar 15;124(6):1404-8.

27 Azémar M, Hildenbrand B, Haering B, Heim ME, Unger C, *Clinical Benefit in Patients with Advanced Solid Tumours Treated with Modified Citrus Pectin: A Prospective Pilot Study.* Clinical Medicine: Oncology 2007:173–80.

28 Jackson CL, Dreaden TM, Theobald LK, Tran NM, Beal TL, Eid M, Gao MY, Shirley RB, Stoffel MT, Kumar MV, Mohnen D, *Pectin induces apoptosis in human prostate cancer cells: correlation of apoptotic function with pectin structure.* Glycobiology 2007;17(8):805-19.

29 Talcott ST, Howard LR, Brenes CH, *Antioxidant Changes and Sensory Properties of Carrot Puree Processed with and without Periderm Tissue.* J. Agric. Food Chem., 2000, 48 (4), pp 1315–1321.

30 Miglio C, Chiavaro E, Visconti A, Fogliano V, Pellegrini N, *Effects of Different Cooking Methods on Nutritional and Physicochemical Characteristics of Selected Vegetables.* J. Agric. Food Chem., 2008, 56 (1), pp 139–147.

31 Dewanto V, Wu X, Adom KK, RH Liu, *Thermal Processing Enhances the Nutritional Value of Tomatoes by Increasing Total Antioxidant Activity.* J. Agric. Food Chem., 2002, 50 (10), pp 3010–3014.

32 Garcia AL, Koebnick C, Dagnelie PC, Strassner C, Elmadfa I, Katz N, Leitzmann C, Hoffmann I, *Long-term strict raw food diet is associated with favourable plasma beta-carotene and low plasma lycopene concentrations in Germans.* Br J Nutr. 2008 Jun;99(6):1293-300.

33 After: Heber, D, *What Color is Your Diet?* HarperCollins, 2001.

34 This table is based on UK National Health Service Guidelines. http://www.5aday.nhs.uk/WhatCounts/PortionSizes.aspx

35 Kaefer CM, Milner JA, *The role of herbs and spices in cancer prevention.* J Nutr Biochem 2008;19(6):347-361. 36 Fang J,

Zhou Q, Liu LZ, *Apigenin inhibits tumour angiogenesis through decreasing HIF-1 and VEGF expression.* Carcinogenesis. 2007 Apr;28(4):858-64.

37 Aggarwal BB, Kunnumakkara AB, Kuzhuvelil B, *Potential of spice-derived phytochemicals for cancer prevention.* Planta Med 2008;74;1560-1569.

38 Craig W, *Health-promoting properties of common herbs.* Am J Clin Nutr 1999;70(s9ppl):419-9S.

39 Shoba G, Joy D, Joseph T, *Influence of piperine on the pharmacokinetics of curcumin in humans and animal volunteers.* Planta Med 1998;64;353-6.

40 Khor TO, Keum YS, Lin W, Kim JH, Hul R, Shen G, Xul C, Gopalakrishnan A, Reddy B, Zheng X, Conney AH, Kong AN, *Combined Inhibitory Effects of Curcumin and Phenethyl Isothiocyanate on the Growth of Human PC-3 Prostate Xenografts in Immunodeficient Mice.* Cancer Research. 2006 Jan; 66(2): 613-621. 2006. PMID:16423986.

41 Cruz-Correa M, Shoskes DA, Sanchez P, Hylind LM, *Combination treatment with curcumin and quercetin of adenomas in familial adenomatous polyposis.* Clin Gastroenterol Hepatol 2006; 4(8):1035-8.

42 Park SY, Murphy SP, Wilkens LR, Henderson BE, Kolonel LN, *Pulse and isoflavone intake and prostate cancer risk: The Multiethnic Cohort Study.* Int J Cancer. 2008 Aug 15;123(4):927-32.

43 Wu AH, Yu MC, Tseng C-C, Pike MC, *Epidemiology of soy exposures and breast cancer risk.* British Journal of Cancer 2008;98:9-14.

44 Shu XO, Zheng Y, Cai H, *Soy food intake and breast cancer survival.* JAMA 2009;302(22):2437-2443.

44a Demark-Wahnefried W, Polascik TJ, George SL et al; *Flaxseed Supplementation (Not Dietary Fat Restriction) Reduces Prostate Cancer Proliferation Rates in Men Presurgery.* Cancer Epidemiol Biomarkers Prev. 2008 Dec;17(12):3577-87.

45 Kuijsten A, Arts ICW, van't Veer P, *The relative bioavailability of enterolignans in humans is enhanced by milling and crushing of flaxseed.* J Nutr 2005 Dec;135(12):2812-6.

46 *Flax seed – storage and baking stability* in *Flax Seed and Human Nutrition*, http://www.flaxcouncil.ca/english/ pdf/stor.pdf

47 Drewnowski A, *Concept of a nutritious food: towards a nutrient density score.* American Journal of Clinical Nutrition 2005. 82(4):721-732.

48 Cordain L, http://www.thepaleodiet.com/faqs/#Fiber; retrieved 4 May 2010

49 Freeman HJ, *Malignancy in adult celiac disease.* World J Gastroenterol. 2009;15(13):1581-1583.

50 Liljeberg H, Bjorck I, *Delayed gastric emptying rate may explain improved glycaemia in healthy subjects to a starchy meal with added vinegar.* Eur J Clin Nutr. 1998 May;52(5):368-71.

51 Liljeberg HG, Lonner CH, Bjorck IM. *Sourdough fermentation or addition of organic acids or corresponding salts to bread improves nutritional properties of starch in healthy humans.* J Nutr. 1995 Jun;125(6):1503-11.

52 See GI/GL database on www.glycemicindex.com

53 Bogdanov S, Jurendic, Sieber R, Gallmann P, *Honey for Nutrition and Health: a Review.* American Journal of the College of Nutrition, 2008, 27: 677-689.

54 Liu H, Huang D, McArthur DL et al, *Fructose induces transketolase flux to promote pancreatic cancer growth.* Cancer Research 2010 Aug 1;70(15):6368-76.

55 Fielding JM, Rowley KG, Cooper P, O' Dea K, *Increases in plasma lycopene concentration after consumption of tomatoes cooked with olive oil.* Asia Pac J Clin Nutr. 2005;14(2):131-6.

56 Brown MJ, Ferruzzi MG, Nguyen ML, Cooper DA, Eldridge AL, Schwartz SJ, White WS, *Carotenoid bioavailability is higher from salads ingested with full-fat than with fat-reduced salad dressings as measured with electrochemical detection.* Am J Clin Nutr. 2004 Aug;80(2):396-403.

57 Waterman E, Lockwood B, *Active components and clinical applications of olive oil.* Alt Med Rev 2007;12(4);331-342.

58 Data from the USDA Nutrient Data Laboratory; Table 3 in Kris-Etherton PM, Harris WS, Appel LJ. *Fish consumption, fish oil, omega-3 fatty acids and cardiovascular disease.* Circulation 2002;106(21):2747-57. The intakes of fish given are very rough estimates because oil content may vary markedly with species, season, diet, and packaging and cooking methods.

59 Huang X, Hites RA, Foran JA, Hamilton C, Knuth BA, Schwager SJ, Carpenter DO, *Consumption advisories for salmon based on risk of cancer and noncancer health effects.* Environ Res. 2006 Jun;101(2):263-74.

60 Corder R, *The Wine Diet.* Sphere 2007.

61 Ramljak D, Romanczyk LJ, Metheney-Barlow LJ, Dickson RB, *Pentameric procyanidin from Theobroma cacao selectively inhibits growth of human breast cancer cells.* Mol Cancer Ther 2005:4(4):537-546.

62 Bisson JF, Guardia-Llorens MA, Hidalgo S, *Protective effect of Acticoa powder, a cocoa polyphenolic extract, on prostate carcinogenesis in Wistar-Unilever rats.* Eur J Cancer Prev. 2008 Feb;17(1):54-61

63 Di Giuseppe R, Di CA, Centritto F, *Regular consumption of dark chocolate is associated with low serum concentrations of C-reactive protein in a healthy Italian population.* J Nutr 2008; 138:1939-1945.

64 Neilson A, George JC, Janle EM, Ferruzzi MG, *Influence of chocolate matrix composition on cocoa flavan-3-ol bioaccessibility in vitro and bioavailability in humans.* J Agric Food Chem 2009, 57, 9418–9426

65 Neilson A, George JC, Janle EM, Ferruzzi MG, *Influence of chocolate matrix composition on cocoa flavan-3-ol bioaccessibility in vitro and bioavailability in humans.* J Agric Food Chem 2009, 57, 9418–9426

66 Stahl L, Miller KB, Apgar J, *Preservation of cocoa antioxidant activity, total polyphenols, flavan-3-ols, and proanthocyanidin content in foods prepared with cocoa powder.* J Food Science 2009;74(6):456-461.

67 Moorman PG, Terry PD, *Consumption of dairy products and the risk of breast cancer: a review of the literature.* Am J Clin Nutr 2004;80:5–14.

68 Swagerty DL, Walling AD, Klein RM, *Lactose Intolerance.* Am Fam Phys 2002;65(9):1845-1850.

69 *Portnoi PA, MacDonald A,* Determination of the lactose and galactose content of cheese for use in the galactosaemia diet. *J Hum Nutr Diet. 2009 Oct;22(5):400-8.*

70 Haenlein GFW, citing Posati & Orr 1976, *Nutritional Value Of Dairy Products Of Ewe And Goat Milk.* 2002. http://goatconnection.com/articles/publish/ article_74.shtml

71 WCRF/AICR, *Food, Nutrition, Physical Activity and the Prevention of Cancer: a Global Perspective.* Washington DC 2007.

72 Environmental Working Group, *Bottled water contains disinfection byproducts, fertilizer residue, and pain medication.* October 2008. http://www.ewg.org/reports/Bottled Water/Bottled-Water-Quality-Investigation, consulted 27 May 2010.

73　Thring TS, Hili P, Naughton DP, *Anti-collagenase, antielastase and anti-oxidant activities of extracts from 21 plants.* BMC Complement Altern Med. 2009 Aug 4;9:27.

74　Carlson JR, Bauer BA, Vincent A, *Reading the tea leaves: anticarcinogenic properties of epigallocatechin-3-gallate.* Mayo Clin Proc 207;82(6): 725-732.

75　Mei Y, Qian F, Wei D, *Reversal of cancer multidrug resistance by green tea polyphenols.* J Pharm Pharmacol. 2004;56(10):1307-14.

76　Sugiyama T, Sadzuka Y, *Theanine, a specific glutamate derivative in green tea, reduces the adverse reactions of doxorubicin by changing the glutathione level.* Cancer Lett. 2004;212(2):177-84.

77　Béliveau R, Gingras D, *Foods to fight cancer: essential foods to help prevent cancer.* Dorling Kindersley, 2007; p. 113.

78　U.S. Department of Agriculture Database for the Flavonoid Content of Selected Foods, http://www.nal. usda.gov/fnic/foodcomp/Data/Flav/Flav02-1.pdf

79　Peters C, Green RJ, Janle EM, Ferruzzi MG, *Formulation with ascorbic acid and sucrose modulates catechin bioavalability from green tea.* Food Res Intl 2010 (43): 95-102.

80　Jansen MC, Bueno-de-Mesquita HB, Feskens EJ, Streppel MT, Kok FJ, Kronhout D, *Quantity and variety of fruit and vegetable consumption and cancer risk.* Nutrition and Cancer 2004;48(2):142-148.

81　Garavetto W, Giordano L, Bosetti C, Talamini R, Negri E, Tavain A, et al, *Diet diversity and the risk of oral and pharyngeal cancer.* Eur J Nutr 2008;47:280-284.

82　La Vecchia C, Munoz SE, Braga C, Fernandez E, Decarli A, *Diet diversity and gastric cancer.* Int J Cancer 1997;72(2):255-7.

83　Lucenteforte E, Garavello W, Bosetti C, Talamini R, Zambon P, Franceschi S, et al, *Diet diversity and the risk of squamous cell esophageal cancer.* Int J Cancer 2008;123:2397-2400.

84　Fernandez E, D'Avanzo B, Negri E, Franceschi S, La Vecchia C, *Diet diversity and the risk of colorectal cancer in northern Italy.* Cancer Epidemiol Biomarkers Prev 1996 Jun;5(6):433-6.

85　Ghadirian P, Narod S, Fafard E, Costa M, Robidoux A, Nkondjock A, *Breast cancer risk in relation to the joint effect of BRCA mutations and diet diversity.* Breast Cancer Res Treat 2009 Jan 23.

86　Michels KB, Wolk A, *A prospective study of variety of healthy foods and mortality in women.* Int J Epidemiol 2002 Aug ;31(4): 847-54.

87　Canene-Adams K, Lindshield BL, Wang S, *Combinations of tomato and broccoli enhance antitumor activity in Dunning R3327-H prostate adenocarcinomas.* Cancer Res 2007;67 (2):836-843.

88　Jian L, Lee AH, Binns CW, *Tea and lycopene protect against prostate cancer.* Asia Pac J Clin Nutr 2007;16(Suppl 1):453-457.

89　Tang FY, Cho HJ, Pai MH, Chen YH, *Concomitant supplementation of lycopene and eicosapentaenoic acid inhibits the proliferation of human colon cancer cells.* J Nutr Biochem. *2009 Jun;20(6):426-34.*

90　Ghadirian P, Narod S, Fafard E, Costa M, Robidoux A, Nkondjock A, *Breast cancer risk in relation to the joint effect of BRCA mutations and diet diversity. Breast Cancer Res Treat 2009.*

91　WCRF/AICR, *Food, Nutrition, Physical Activity and the Prevention of Cancer: a Global Perspective.* Washington DC, 2007.

92　Motallebnejad M, Akram S, Moghadamnia A, Moulana Z, Omidi S, *The effect of topical application of pure honey on radiation-induced mucositis: a randomized clinical trial.* J Contemp Dental Practice 2008 (9)3: 40-47.

93　Bardy J, Slevin NJ, Mais KL, Molassiotis A, *A systematic review of honey uses and its potential value within oncology care.* J Clin Nurs. *2008 Oct;17(19):2604-23.*

Chapter 5

1　Beck, ME, Dinner preparation in the modern United States. British Food Journal 2007, 109(7); 531-547.

1a　Fiese BH, Winter MA, Botti JC, *The ABCs of family mealtimes: Observational lessons for promoting healthy outcomes for children with persistent asthma.* Child Development 2011 (83)1; 133-145.

2　Goulet J, Lamarche B, Lemieux S, *A nutritional intervention promoting a Mediterranean food pattern does not affect total dietary cost in North American women in free-living conditions.* Journal of Nutrition 2008; 138: 54-59.

3　What Consumer, October 31, 2008, http:// whatconsumer. co.uk/food-money-saving-study/

General index *(for recipes, see **Recipe index** p. 278)*

Recipe index

CPSIA information can be obtained at www.ICGtesting.com
Printed in the USA
LVOW090908060912

297466LV00004B/208/P